GET FIREFIGHTER FIT

GET FIREFIGHTER FIT

The Complete Workout from the Former Director of the New York City Fire Department Physical Training Program

KEVIN S. MALLEY
DAVID K. SPIERER

photographs by William Wittkop

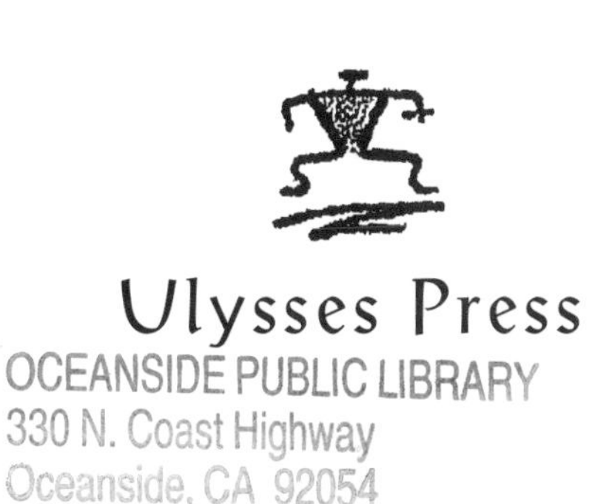

Ulysses Press

Published in the United States by
ULYSSES PRESS
P.O. Box 3440
Berkeley, CA 94703
www.ulyssespress.com

ISBN10: 1-56975-626-0
ISBN13: 978-1-56975-626-3
Library of Congress Control Number 2007905321

Printed in Canada by Webcom

10 9 8 7 6 5 4 3 2 1

Acquisitions	Nick Denton-Brown
Editorial/Production	Lily Chou, Claire Chun, Lauren Harrison, Judith Metzener, Steven Schwartz
Index	Sayre Van Young
Cover design	what!design @ whatweb.com
Cover photography	© iStockphoto.com/Les Byerley (front) and © iStockphoto.com/Sille Van Landschoot (back)
Models	Erin Bradley, Dane Coleman, Alex Hamburger, Charles Healey, Felix Reyes, Deblin Rodriguez, William Sinnott, Daniel Sullivan, Richie Velez, Sergio Villamizar, Anthony Wolleon
Interior photographs	William Wittkop except p. vi © Joan M. Malley; p. 5 © iStockphoto.com/Sabina Salihbasic; p. 10 © iStockphoto.com/Craig Robinson; p. 13 © Edward McCauley; p. 20 © iStockphoto.com/Diego Cervo; p. 24 © photos.com; p. 30 © iStockphoto.com/Xavi Arnau; p. 53 © The New York City Fire Department; page 57 © The New York City Fire Department

Distributed by Publishers Group West

Please Note
This book has been written and published strictly for informational purposes, and in no way should be used as a substitute for actual instruction with qualified professionals. The authors and publisher are providing you with information in this work so that you can have the knowledge and can choose, at your own risk, to act on that knowledge. The authors and publisher also urge all readers to be aware of their health status and to consult health care professionals before beginning any health or exercise program.

This book is dedicated to the fallen firefighters and fire officers with whom I had the great honor and privilege of working and/or training with through my term as a firefighter and fire officer with the New York City Fire Department. These men, in the most honorable tradition of our profession, gave so much of themselves in their commitment to assist others in need. Their contributions were as immeasurable as the loss we continue to feel in their absence:

Thomas Gardner, Kevin Donnelly, Peter McLaughlin, Scott LaPiedra, Patrick Brown, John McAvoy, William McGinn, Ronald P. Bucca, Edward F. Geraghty, Dennis Cross, Thomas Foley, Thomas T. Haskell, Jr., Robert Hamilton, Donald J. Regan, Vernon A. Richard, Timothy Stackpole, John M. Paolillo, William M. Feehan, Peter Ganci, Raymond M. Downey, Terrence S. Hatton, Christopher Blackwell, Charles J. Margiotta, Charles L. Casper, Lawrence T. Stack, Jonathan L. Ielpi, Michael Mullen, Lawrence J. Virgillio, Hector I. Tirado, Jr., John P. Williamson, Christopher A. Santora, Timothy S. Haskell, Michael Boyle, William F. Burke, Jr., Charles Garbarini, James R. Coyle, Dennis Devlin, Jeffrey J. Giordano, Vincent F. Giammona, Thomas Kelly, Michael V. Kiefer and ("young") Dave Farrell.

Acknowledgments

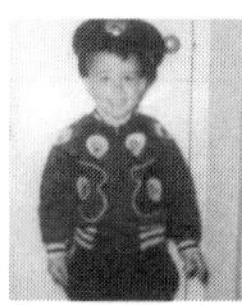
Thanks, Smokey

We would like to thank the following individuals and organizations for their gracious contributions and assistance in the completion of this book: Dr. William D. McArdle, Dr. Eric Malmberg, Daniel Caffrey, Richard Nagel, Michael Andreachi, Thomas Grimshaw, Jan Schlegel, Mark Cohen, Sergio Villamizar, James M. Roberts, Michael Scaniello, George Deaver, Ellen Wayman-Gordon, New Jersey City University, and the fire departments of Milburn and South Orange, New Jersey.

Table of Contents

Introduction

In the spring of 1996, the recently appointed commissioner of the New York City Fire Department, Thomas Von Essen, offered me a newly created position as the director of human performance. During our interview, he stated that if I were to accept the position, he would provide me with the support I needed to develop any conceivable program that might potentially improve the health, safety and performance of New York City firefighters. I accepted the offer and, for a period of slightly more than five years, worked together with an extraordinary group of dedicated colleagues (including the inexhaustible Dr. David J. Penzant) on a broad variety of projects in nearly every branch of the department. We worked tirelessly, committed to "giving back to the job" we all felt so strongly about and absolutely believed in, trying to do whatever we could to make "our job" (FDNY firefighting) a better and safer occupation for all those currently in the field as well as those who were yet to come.

Receiving unprecedented support from the commissioner and his administration, as well as key support from the unions, we worked within the department and also partnered with the New York State Division of Fire Prevention and Control, the International Association of Fire Fighters (IAFF) and International Association of Fire Chiefs (IAFC) to develop health and fitness programs for firefighters in New York City, New York State and across the nation. Most importantly, as a consequence of the committed efforts of a sensational staff led by FDNY unit directors Patrick McFadden and Michael Cacciola, we created a full spectrum of successful physical training programs for FDNY firefighters, fire officers, alumni, Emergency Medical Service (EMS) personnel, firefighter cadets, civilian staff, and FDNY candidates. Additionally, we contributed to the IAFF/IAFC Wellness Initiative, Candidate Physical Ability Test (CPAT) and Peer Fitness Trainer Program.

This book was written with the same intention and philosophy as most, if not all, of our previous work—that is, to enable motivated people like you to train and achieve the peak level of fitness exhibited by high-performance firefighters. As with our previous efforts, this book will provide you with the tools and direction you need to improve your personal fitness, health and either athletic or fireground performance and safety. Dave and I have combined our diverse academic, professional and athletic experiences to produce a unique and effective training tool. Having trained literally thousands of incumbent and prospective firefighters as well as EMS workers, civilians and college athletes, we recognize absolutely the importance of communicating clearly in order to facilitate learning and optimize training results.

Whether you're a civilian, athlete, or prospective or incumbent firefighter, you will see, learn and understand how every aspect of your training relates directly to the development of your fitness capacities and high-intensity physical performance.

The photographic support of exercise descriptions will enable you to make the direct connection between a multitude of firefighting tasks and the specific exercises you perform. As you execute each repetition of your exercise sets, envision yourself completing real firefighting tasks. You will in essence be the firefighter, forcing open doors and extinguishing rooms of fire. This is the way to stay focused and maintain a high level of motivation throughout the course of your training. This is the way to achieve the greatest gains and train most effectively for high performance on the athletic field or in the field of fire. This is the way to *Get Firefighter Fit*.

Good luck with your training, and may you enjoy the conditioning process as well as the improvements that result.

Kevin S. Malley
Jersey City, New Jersey
May 2008

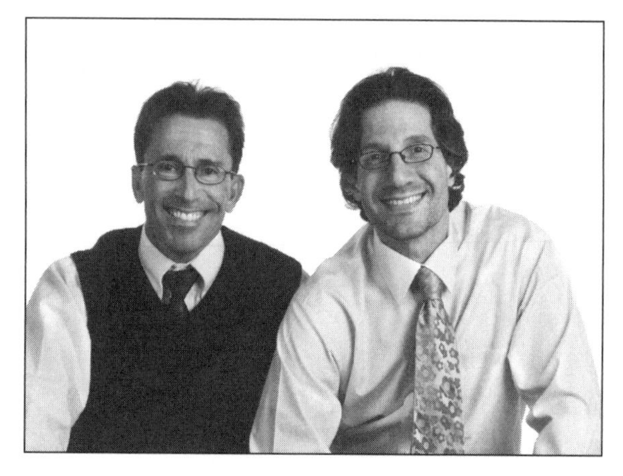

Authors Kevin Malley (left) and David Spierer

You Are the Firefighter

It's almost nine o'clock. Your day tour is about to begin.

After two cups of coffee, a bagel and 30 minutes of banter with the crew, you slip out of the kitchen to check out the rig. It's a beautiful summer day. As you walk onto the apparatus floor, a warm, familiar sensation arises in your gut. The scent of last night's fire is in the air.

You glance at the crew's gear and then move toward the rig. Your eyes focus and affix on the ornate lettering of the aerial ladder: Ladder Company 40. You don't have to think about it—you feel it and you just know it, deep inside. This is where you want to be. This is what you want to do. You're a firefighter and you serve to save other people's lives. This is the greatest job.

Knowing that preparation is the key to success in any athletic activity, you begin each tour of duty by inspecting your gear and tools. This equipment enables high-level performance and can save your life. You remove your protective turnout coat and pants, helmet and boots from the rack. They feel a little heavy this morning, still damp from yesterday's fire. You rummage through the coat pockets, checking for gloves, hood, knife and other personal equipment. No wonder the gear weighs so much. The jacket's only about 40 pounds out of the box, but certainly much heavier today, dirty, wet and loaded with tools. You lay out the gear by your riding position, organizing it so you can dress quickly in response to an alarm.

Stepping up on the rig's side running board, you open the passenger compartment door and move inside. You place your helmet, hood and flashlight on the engine compartment beside your seat, and then turn and grab hold of the shoulder harness straps of your air mask. One forceful pull with one arm frees the 30-pound mask from its brackets. It's kind of a cumbersome piece of equipment but worth its weight in gold at a fire. Cool, clean air in a super-heated and toxic environment is priceless—it's your lifeline. Heart disease and cancer prevail among those who have worked without it.

Being assigned to the forcible-entry team "can" position, you inspect your designated tools: a six-foot wood and metal hook and a two-and-a-half-gallon water extinguisher. You lift the can from its holder and note by its weight that it's full. Still, you check the pressure gauge to make sure. It's in the green, you're good to go. Lugging 30 pounds of water in a metal can may be a pain in the butt at times, but when you need it to contain a growing fire so that you can make a quick search or rescue, you wish you had two.

Next you inspect the two power saws. You lift them out of the compartment one at a time. Each saw weighs about 25 pounds. Is every piece of equipment on this rig another 25 to 30 pounds? You smile as you realize the answer to your own question: The portable ladders weigh between 65 and 110 pounds, depending on their length.

Securing the saw with your left hand and foot and grasping the starting cord handle firmly with your right, you pull upward in one powerful stroke. The engine kicks over and soars into a deafening roar. As you rev the saw up to full throttle, you can just barely hear the incoming alarm. You quickly remove your finger from the throttle and shut off the saw. Alarm lights illuminate, apparatus doors begin to rise and the house watchman commands over the intercom, "Everybody get out, all companies respond!"

The firehouse comes to life. Firefighters run toward the fire engines from all directions, slide down poles from the second floor and burst out of the kitchen. You hustle to get the saws back into the compartment on the rig, slam the door shut, check that it's locked and then bolt over to your gear. As you kick off your shoes and slide into your pants, you focus intensely on two key objectives: dressing swiftly and listening for any additional information coming over the PA. The emergency lights on the rig suddenly activate and the motor roars to life. As you throw on your coat and jump on board, you hear the house watchman's parting announcement, "Reported building fire at 12 West 9th Street, apartment 5A as in Adam!"

You pull up your hood, secure your coat and then roll up and fasten your collar. You don your helmet, switch on your radio and slip into the arm straps of your mask. Finally you clip on your flashlight and reach for your gloves. The seatbelt is too tight. You're packed in between the engine compartment and side wall of the cab like a sardine. The noise of the accelerating diesel motor is overbearing and you strain to hear the anticipated radio communications of the fire department dispatcher and other responding units. Any additional information helps.

A bead of sweat trickles down your face and drops onto your lap. Your shirt is already clinging to your skin. The gear is great protection from burns, cuts, abrasions and toxic exposures but, man, does it make you sweat! Water or juice rather than coffee would've been the smarter move this morning. You're dressed like a mummy and sweating like a hog, two further challenges with which you'll have to contend.

"Manhattan dispatch to all responding units, we're receiving numerous phone calls for box 714, reported address 12 West 9th Street. Be advised there are reports of people trapped in apartment 5A on the fifth floor."

Your heart is pounding through your chest. Anticipation and bridled fear inspire the sensation of butterflies in your gut. This is your fire, you're first due. You have to get up there, force that door, locate any victims and get them out. Time is of the essence. Seconds seem like minutes. The ladder company's siren wails and air horn blasts as the chauffeur weaves around, past and through the busy city streets.

With your ear pressed against the speaker of your portable radio, you strain to hear the critical communications of the officer and other members of the first arriving engine. You try to recall and envision the physical features of the reported fire building. You've been down that street a thousand times. What does the building look like? How tall, wide and deep is it? What are the apartment layouts? Where are the bedrooms? Are there any fire escapes? Your mind is racing. Sweat runs down your forehead, into your eyes. You wipe it with your hood.

Suddenly, a rapid series of communications are made between the officer of the first due Engine Company and the Fire Department dispatcher. "Engine 37 to Manhattan, go ahead, Engine 37."

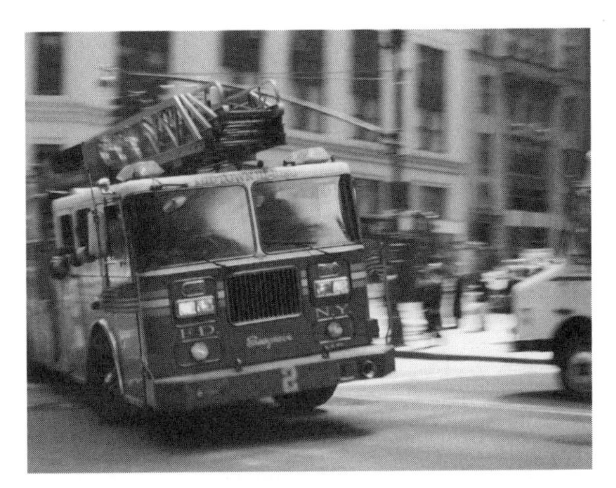

"Ten-eighty-four at box 714, 10-75."

For a fraction of a second your world stands still. It's confirmed you've got a "job." The butterflies in your stomach take flight again and soar.

The dialog between the officer and the fire department dispatch continue. "We have a working fire in an occupied five-story, non-fireproof multiple dwelling. Fire is venting out three windows on the top floor, exposure one side of the building 'K.'"

"Ten-four, Engine 37."

You run the initial size-up through your mind, developing an effective plan of action. "Three windows of fire. That means two or more rooms are already involved and the fire is likely extending. We'll need to get up there fast. Fire is on the top floor, which means there's nowhere for the heat, smoke and fire to go. It's going to be hot and there's a good chance the fire will spread up above the ceiling and across the top floor. Visibility will be zero and fire could light up almost anywhere. It's going to be extremely dangerous—hot, smoky and potentially explosive. Easy to get disorienated, trapped or killed. We better work quick and smart."

The rig brakes to a sudden halt and you're on the scene. Your colleague swings open the cab door and ejects from the rig. You exit right behind. In one swift set of movements you grab your hook and extinguisher and bolt toward the building. Your officer is five feet ahead. He glances over his shoulder to make sure you're close behind. You're walking at a cadence just short of a run.

Chaos reigns. People are fleeing, crying and screaming, in varied states of horror, shock and pain. Sirens wail and air horns blast, rig doors spring open and additional firefighters jump out. Directions are being issued and commands are being made. As the firefighters move in, terrified civilians scramble frantically out and away.

You maneuver erratically toward the building through a crowd of spectators and evacuating residents. Filtering out the overpowering distractions as best you can, you attempt to stay calm, cool and collected. You take in as much important information as you can without getting too emotionally involved. The drama associated with such catastrophic events can be overwhelming, especially for new recruits, but you can't let it distract or deter you. Fear, anxiety and pain are unavoidable consequences of the job. The key is to learn how to see through the chaos, recognize the dangers and use the critical information you collect to get the job done.

Approaching the building rapidly, you continue to gather information and piece together the fire situation. "One, two, three, four, five stories. Fire is out three windows on the top floor and heavy smoke is pushing out of the cornice seams. The fire has gotten a good foot hold and is likely spreading fast. No fire escape in the front and six windows on each floor. That means there's probably a fire escape in the rear if we need it and two apartments running front to rear on each floor. The buildings to each side are attached, of similar construction and dimensions, and occupied. Potential exposure problems and life hazard if the fire continues to extend."

Suddenly, a man yells, "There's a woman up there with a baby."

You look up. A woman's head is sticking out a top-floor window adjacent to the windows venting heavy fire and black smoke. She's screaming, but you can't make out what she's saying with all of the noise. Five stories up—if she jumps, she's dead.

She's holding a baby and leans out the window. It's too high for a portable ladder and the electrical wires in the street may make it impossible to get her with the aerial ladder. You have got to get up there fast! You're their only prospect for survival.

Banging into one person after another, you fight to make your way toward the building's entrance. Breaching through the bottleneck of evacuees, you enter the building and accelerate like a running back having just busted through the line. Charging for the stairs, you're emotionally psyched. The absolute urgency of the situation is nearly overwhelming. The clock is running. You know the consequences of delay. Seconds will mean the difference between life and death.

As you hit the stairs, you're right on your officer's back. This is why you bike five days a week. Your fitness enables you to ascend the five flights of stairs as quickly as possible. You can't afford to be exhausted when you get there. There are no breaks on the fire floor, no time-outs to recover from the climb. As soon as you get there, you have to go right to work. You have to locate the fire apartment, force open the door, find those two people and get them out to the paramedics *alive*.

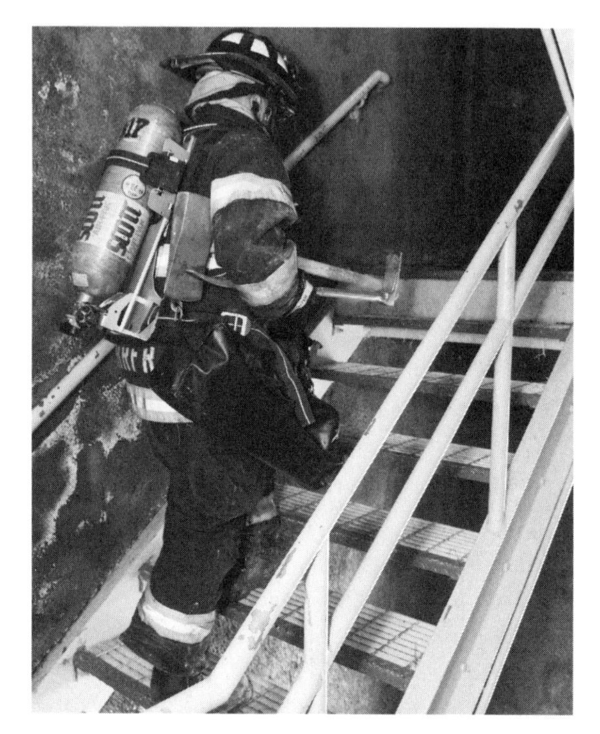

The protective clothing, equipment and tools that you shoulder weigh in excess of 110 pounds. Friction, restriction and heat stress from the encapsulating clothing further impact your every step and stride. By the time you reach the third floor, your quads are burning and your lungs heave with each accelerated breath. You've lost a step or two on your officer but are still pretty close behind. Of course he's a little quicker. He's only carrying a two-pound plastic flashlight and a kid-size crowbar.

You concentrate on the stairs, pumping your legs like pistons and pulling yourself up with the banister. At the turn of the third-floor landing, you see your partner in close pursuit. He's breathing pretty heavy, too, but he still looks strong, pushing off the balls of his feet. He'll make it no problem, he's a runner.

Leaning forward into the stairs, you vigorously pound out the last two flights of your ascent. The dialog between your officer and the operations chief inspire you to pick up the pace.

"Battalion 7 to Ladder 40, are you up there yet?"

"Ladder 40 to Battalion, we're almost there, Chief."

"Ladder 40, be advised we are unable to get to the woman and child from the outside. The aerial is blocked out by overhead wires. We've got a life-saving rope en route to the roof, but the second-due ladder company is delayed. Let me know if you guys can get to them from the inside. Let me know what's going on when you get in there."

"Ladder 40, 10-4."

High levels of adrenaline and lactic acid flow through your body as a consequence of the intense physical and psychological stresses. You begin to feel nauseous. It's a good thing you had a bagel instead of the fried eggs and pig's butt this morning. No cramps, and the bagel is less likely to come up.

You yank on the banister and push through the pain as you surge up the final ten steps. Your quads scream and lungs sear as your heart thunders through your breastbone. Three, two, one, you're there!

The landing is filled with smoke. You instinctively hit the floor and crawl toward your officer. He's kneeling beside the apartment door, donning his mask. Still breathing heavily and coughing from the acrid smoke, you remove your gloves and helmet to do the same. Your partner goes directly to the door. As you pull up your protective hood and throw on your helmet, you see your officer getting control of the door. He grabs a hold of the knob with one hand, checking to see if it's locked. Simultaneously, he slides his other hand across the upper regions to see if the door's hot. He quickly issues concise directions, "Steel door—steel frame with multiple locks engaged. No heat, let's force it."

You pick up the six-pound maul and your partner places his steel Halligan tool into place. The officer maintains control of the door with his hose strap and shines his flashlight on the locks you're about to attack. There's so much smoke it's almost impossible to see the door. You position yourself so that you can swing the maul powerfully and precisely through a consistent plane. Your partner yells, "Hit!"

Crouched in a stable and power-generating stance, you act in one explosive and coordinated movement, rotating your trunk, slightly extending your right arm and pushing forward with your back leg. *Boom!* The Halligan hardly moves. The door is going to be tough.

Your partner shouts "Hit" again and again. Each time he barks, you forcefully strike with your maul. The thunder of pounding steel echoes loudly in the hallway. Every muscle group is engaged as you stabilize your power position and repeatedly exert near-maximal force. You've been working for a

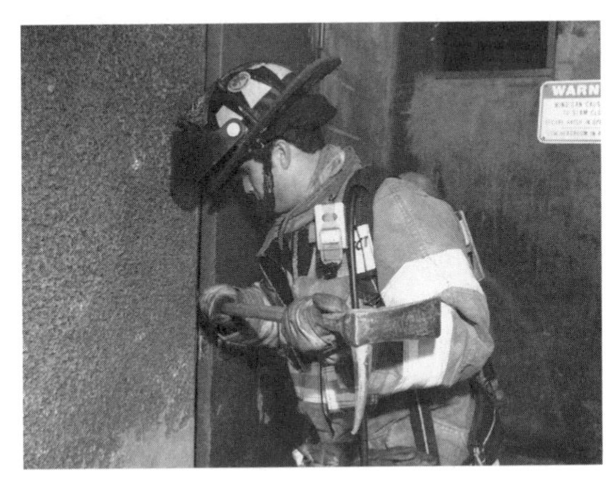

minute but it seems like much longer. Your arms are beginning to fatigue, but you can't slow down—it's just *not* an option.

Finally, you feel the Halligan start to give. The fork starts to make its way into the seam of the door. This has to be the fifteenth shot. You strike it one more time.

Your partner yells, "I think we got it!"

The fork is in past the door frame. He leans on the Halligan to pry the door open. A radio transmission breaks in. It's the chief calling for an update.

"Any progress up there, Ladder 40? We've lost sight of the woman and child. They're no longer at the window."

With that, the door pops free of the frame. The officer keeps it shut with his hose strap until he completes his communication to the chief. "Ladder 40 to Battalion 7, we have the door forced and we're going in."

You hand the maul to your partner, grab your hook and extinguisher and move right behind your officer. Nervous, pumped and intensely focused, you anticipate the dangerous actions you're about to take. The environment will be absolutely lethal: toxic, severely heated and potentially explosive.

Your officer grabs the doorknob and releases his hose strap. He cracks the door open just a hair. Heavy gray and black smoke pushes out from around the top of the door. Seeing no flames, he pushes the door open and moves in. He immediately checks behind the door for victims and then secures it open with a wooden chock. Dragging your water extinguisher and hook, you crawl swiftly to stay on his heels.

Your officer yells out in hopes of a response from the victims, "Fire department, fire department! Where are you? Fire department! Where are you?"

There's no reply. You can't see anything in the heavy smoke.

Maintaining contact with the wall with your left hand, you sweep in front and to the right of you with your hook. Your officer is moving fast and you struggle to stay right with him, searching quickly as you go. It's getting noticeably hotter as you progress deeper into the apartment. Orange flames flicker through the smoke just ahead and to the right. They're surging across the ceiling from an open doorway.

Suddenly, you bang head-on into your officer and fall over. As you scramble back on your knees, he grabs your shoulder and instructs you to use your extinguisher to contain the fire so that he can crawl past it and search the back room.

Getting as low as you can and moving to the side of the doorway to minimize exposure to the flames and severe heat, you direct the stream of water from your extinguisher upward toward the flames. It works to some extent, temporarily pushing the flames back inside the doorway. But it's getting really bad fast and two and a half gallons of water isn't going to buy much time.

You hear your officer yell out from the back room. He's located the woman and child, and you hear his transmission over the radio: "Ladder 40 to Battalion 7, we have two 10-45 code 2s in apartment 5A. A woman and young child. We need a handline up here fast, it's gonna light up!"

They must be unconscious. He's going to need help getting them out. Your partner comes up from behind you, squeezes by and then crawls beneath the fire and past the doorway. Within seconds he returns, crawling rapidly back past the fire. The baby is cradled in his arms. He knocks you over as he barrels past. The extinguisher is ripped from your hands. You quickly grab a hold of it and reapply the stream of water toward the flames. It's not working anymore. The flames are out of the door and rolling over your head. You're almost out of water, exhausted and burning through your gear. You have to get out of here before the apartment "flashes." Where the hell is the officer? You yell out, "Captain, you ok, you need help? I'm almost out of water. The fire is out the door."

Just then you see his helmet. He's moving toward you on the floor. "Give me a hand!"

He's trying to drag the woman out. You drop the near-empty extinguisher and spring past the fire. He pulls her from under her arms and you push from below. Together you strain with all of your might to transport her swiftly down the hallway toward the front door. She's unconscious, heavy and extremely difficult to move. You grunt and grind your teeth as you lift her from the legs and simultaneously push her forward. You cringe from the searing heat as you pass the fire. You keep going. You're absolutely shot, but you keep lifting and pushing, lifting and pushing. Your back aches, your legs burn and your arms are beginning to fail. Where the hell's the door?

The fire is surging down the hallway right behind you. You can feel the intense heat. You're completely exhausted and fighting the overwhelming urge to collapse. You're shouting at yourself in an attempt to win the powerful internal augment that ensues, "Keep going! You can't stop now! This place is going to light up! We have to get out of here! Don't quit! Keep going! Go! Go!"

Your officer shouts, "Come on, just a little more, we're almost there!"

You dig down, and with one last surge, barrel straight ahead and out through the door. You fall over on your side outside the apartment. There are firefighters all around you and a great deal of commotion. You try to get up. Firefighters from the second-due ladder company are lifting the woman off the floor. You hear one firefighter say, "She's breathing. Come on, let's get her downstairs quick!"

Your officer grabs a hold of you and kneels by your side. "You alright, kid?"

You reflexively respond, "I'm OK, Captain. I'm good."

"Nice job. Come on, let's go down to the street."

You roll over and struggle to get up. You grab the railing and slowly pull yourself to your feet. The stairway and landing are now congested with firefighters. The engine company's line is charged with water and they're moving in. Members of the second- and third-due ladder companies are moving past you to finish the job. Using the banister as a crutch, you hobble slowly down the five flights to the street. You're a little shaky. Your legs sting as you bend them, you're burnt. That was a close one. Thank God you're training. You hope the woman and baby make it.

The physical demands of firefighting are comprehensive and severe. To operate effectively under such adverse conditions, firefighters need to be courageous, skilled and highly conditioned. With each response, like a fighter approaching the ring, firefighters know that their performance depends upon their fitness and that at any given time their personal fitness can mean the difference between life and death. That's why so many firefighters are committed to achieving and maintaining a high level of fitness; they know that when they step into the gym, there's a damn good reason for being there. They don't just train for the hell of it, they "train for life."[12]

Whether you're currently "on the job," aspiring to become a firefighter or desire to achieve the fitness level of a high-performance firefighter, your success in training will be to the greatest extent determined by your ability to stay motivated and train smart. Every good coach understands this. Keeping athletes motivated and moving them through a well-balanced personalized training progression optimizes the rate and extent of their development. You've already got the motivation, so now it becomes our job to try and help you to use it in the most productive way and guide you toward the accomplishment of your training goals. Grant us the privilege of coaching you through your training and we'll do our best to assist you in your efforts to achieve the peak fitness level of a high-performance firefighter/athlete.

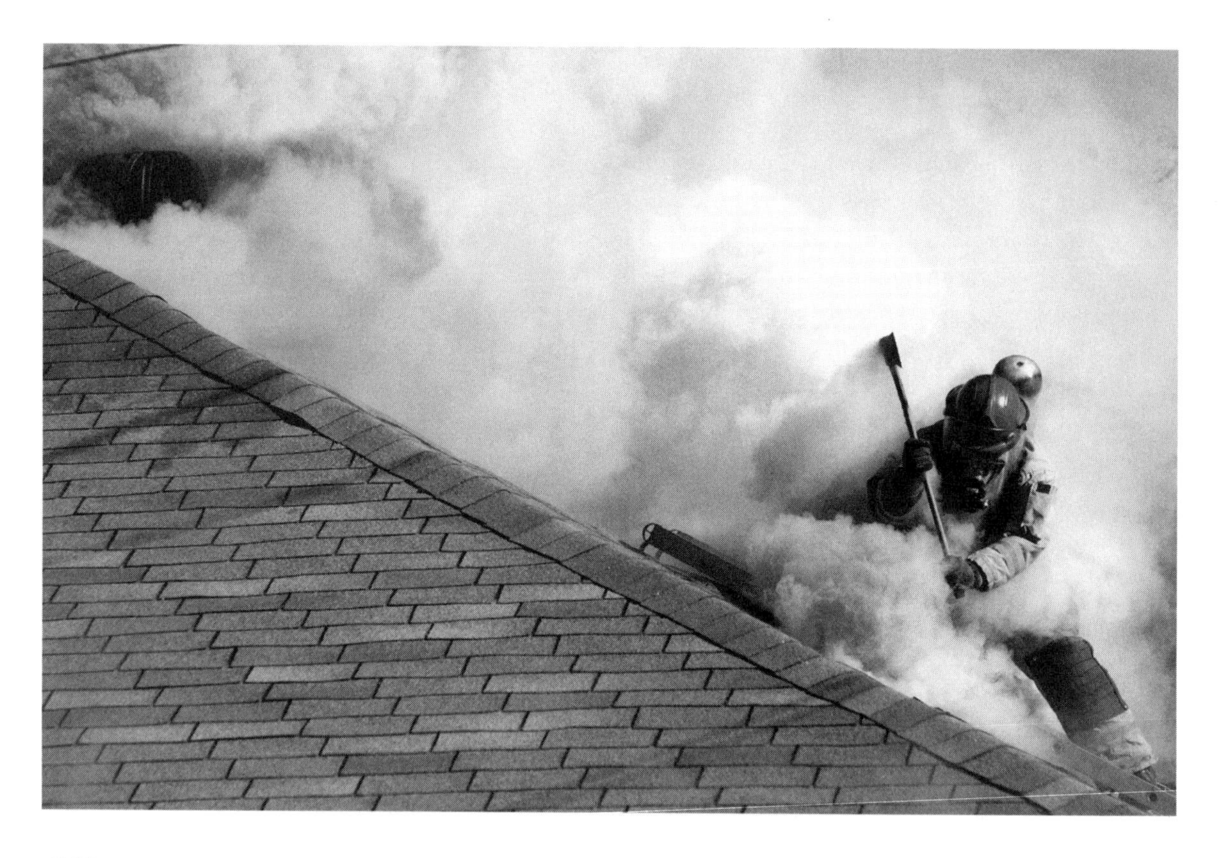

Firefighter Fit Training Principles

Training is a lot like taking your family on vacation. First you decide where you want to go, then you do a little research and map it out. Finally, just before leaving, you get the car thoroughly serviced for the ride. Can you imagine jumping into the car with your wife and kids for a cross-country trip and just trying to wing it? Forget about it—that's a recipe for disaster!

Physical training is essentially the same: If you launch into a physical training program blindly, the prospect for success is remote. No matter how enthusiastic you are at the start, a reckless or haphazard approach to training most often leads to frustration and failure. That's one reason why health clubs experience such a high rate of attrition; people jump in ill prepared and fail within weeks or days. Consider firefighters who arrive at the scene of a horrific fire—if they hop off the fire engine and go charging right into the flaming building, they're destined to make critical mistakes. Avoid this common pitfall. Approach your training like a seasoned traveler or veteran firefighter; decide what you want to do, gather important (training) information, develop an effective (training) strategy and then use it to achieve your (training) goals.

The following sections will provide you with the information you need to identify your primary training goal(s), select the appropriate form(s) of training and develop a well-balanced, progressive training program. Then, all you need to do is make certain you're in good health and away you go. Your success in training lies straight ahead. Just continue to read, use what you learn and train to succeed. Develop your personalized program, commit to the process of gradual, intelligent and progressive training, and then work hard to achieve the peak fitness level of a high-performance firefighter.

STEP 1. Select Your Primary Goal

The first important step in the training process is to clearly define your primary training goal(s). In firefighting, determining the primary goal of an operation is generally quite easy as it almost always centers on the functions of saving lives and/or protecting property. In training, however, the spectrum of primary goals is much broader. This can make the selection process a bit more challenging.

One approach that we've found to be successful in assisting athletes in their efforts to determine their primary training goal(s) is to have them ask themselves a few simple questions. The first, of course, is the classic, "What is it that you *really* want to achieve?" For some people this is a relatively easy question to answer; for others, however, it is not. If the answer doesn't pop right out, don't be alarmed. Just ask yourself a couple of slightly more specific questions, such as: "Are you training to improve your performance in the fire field or to just shed a few unwanted (fat) pounds?" "Do you want to increase your muscular strength, endurance or flexibility, or just look great and feel like an athletic powerhouse?" You get the picture. Narrow down your answer(s) and try to develop one or more clear and achievable goal(s). Once you've done this, you're ready to begin the process of formulating your personalized training program.

STEP 2. Develop Your Personalized Training Program

Having identified one or more primary training goals, your next task is to select the appropriate form(s) of training and specific types of conditioning exercises to enable your targeted development. This is another very important step in the process, so once again give your selections some considerable thought. Remember, each exercise is an important piece of the training puzzle. As you make your selections and piece them together to form creative training routines, you'll observe your personal training strategy coming to life. It's actually pretty exciting work. Good coaches, in particular, love this part of the process.

In terms of your selections, it's important to understand absolutely that the best form of training and type of training exercises for you are those which are most effective at producing the enhancements you desire. Therefore, the type of training that best fits your needs is the one that develops the specific muscles, energy-producing (metabolic) pathways and other systems that you wish to improve. This fundamental training principle is referred to as the "specificity of training." It's so logical a principle that you'd expect everyone to automatically apply it to their training, but in fact many don't. This is one reason why so many hard-working athletes never reach their full potential. You don't want to go down this road. What you're looking for is the greatest return from your training investment. So give your selection of training type some considerable thought. Ideally, you should select a form of training that is both enjoyable and most effective at promoting the type of development you desire. In firefighting, we refer to this as "using the right tool for the job."

As an example, if your primary training goal is to improve the muscular endurance of your legs and thereby your ability to ascend stairs, then you'd want to choose an exercise that utilizes the same muscles you use when climbing stairs. If you're training in a gym that has stepping machines, developing a training program that centers around these would be ideal. Given that many of the same muscles employed in stair climbing are also used with running or cycling, these forms of exercises are also good options.

If you want to increase total body strength and muscular endurance, then resistance training would be the exercise training "tool" of choice. Using moderately heavy weights and completing a relatively higher number of repetitions (15–20) will effectively develop the specific muscles, tissues and systems necessary to increase the amount of force you can produce repeatedly when executing physical tasks. Training specificity is fundamental to optimal training response and development, so in order to realize the most dramatic gains, you must select the correct type(s) of training and then commit to using it/them consistently in a safe and progressive manner. In the Strength Training section ahead, we provide a variety of programs designed to

FIREFIGHTER/ATHLETE PROFILES

Having the good fortune of working with many outstanding firefighter/athletes throughout my career, I have witnessed firsthand the influence of specific forms of training on firefighting performance. In this regard, the field performances of two firefighter/athletes come immediately to mind.

One firefighter, Gary Connolly, was so well conditioned as a cyclist that he could make his way to the roof of a five-story building before the inside team reached the fire floor two or three floors below. Gary would be giving a preliminary report from the roof before the forcible entry team began working on the door of the apartment that was on fire. Firefighter Connolly, like so many other cyclists, always seemed to be the fastest when it came to ascending stairs. The runners were great, but the cyclists were even better. This makes sense, given that the same muscles (quadriceps) serve as the primary movers in both activities.

Another extraordinary firefighter/athlete, Timothy McCauley was a very successful triathlete and competitive runner who conditioned and competed with the same level of expertise and intensity as he did with fighting fires. Late one evening, we responded to a fire where trapped civilians were hanging and jumping from the top-floor windows of a building as we arrived. Tim was the nozzleman of the first-due engine company (Engine 37). It was the kind of fire situation where everything had to be done right—and fast. In a manner of speaking, this is the highest level of the game: urgent, complex and extremely dangerous. Ladder Company 40 went after the trapped civilians from all angles and Lieutenant John Keenan led Engine 37 to the fire. Civilian life hung on the balance, depending solely upon the performance capacities of the responding firefighters. The interior stairway was fully involved with fire, forcing Tim to begin his attack on the fire at the base of the stairs. Opening the nozzle, he pushed the fire back and launched into his ascent. Constantly pushing forward, he just kept knocking the fire down as he crawled up the stairs. He never shut down the nozzle and never stopped moving. Sliding back half the distance he gained with each step, slipping on fallen plaster from the collapsing ceiling above, Tim just kept pushing upward and extinguishing fire. He finally stopped at the top floor, for he had run out of fire. This level of performance doesn't just occur—it requires great effort and training, courage, skill and a very high caliber of fitness. Tim's commitment to swimming, cycling and running translated directly into peak-level, life-saving performance this evening, and enabled him to consistently perform at the highest level throughout the full term of his distinguished firefighting career.

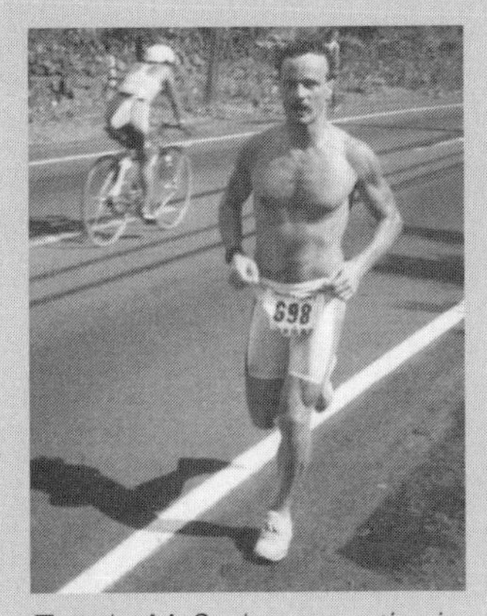

Timothy McCauley competing in the Ironman Triathlon.

assist you in achieving your personal training goals. The diverse focus and flexible design of these programs enable you to create a program that will develop the specific muscles and muscular capacities that you desire (e.g., muscular endurance, strength, size).

The Importance of Training Specificity

Utilizing the principle of training specificity can help firefighters avoid injury as well as optimize the rate in which they develop their physical abilities to perform. We used a progressive form of physical conditioning with entrance-level firefighters in the FDNY Fire Academy that simultaneously cultivated firefighter fitness and job skill performance. We called it "performance training." With this training, firefighters completed a progressive series of increasingly more challenging job tasks. Emphasizing the principle of training specificity, we constantly evaluated a firefighter's ability to successfully complete these critical tasks. If a firefighter struggled with a particular task as a consequence of insufficient strength, muscular endurance or aerobic capacity, they'd be immediately referred to a specialized physical training program. Each program was uniquely designed to improve the specific muscle groups and capacities that enabled the successful completion of the given firefighting task.

STEP 3. Train Consistently

Consistency is the absolute key to training success. As important as all of the other components of your training program may be, the only way that you're going to progress, improve and achieve your training goals is by training on a consistent basis. Somehow you need to find a way to either make or take the time routinely to break loose and get it done. Chances are this won't be easy. In fact, finding the time to train on a given day may be more challenging than the workout itself.

We recommend that you take a good, hard look at your daily schedule. Check to see if there are any routine periods of availability and try to find the most practical and painless way of fitting a brief training session into your daily life. For many people, these intervals of availability wind up being either before work, after work or during lunch. If this is the case with you, then the next logical step is to decide which of these periods is most consistently convenient or the easiest to do. Try to be realistic. If you're not, and your training conflicts with other important priorities (like sleep or dinner with the family), you're doomed to the same fate as the millions who did so before you: failure.

Keep in mind that, as a rule, on any given day there are at least a thousand "good reasons" not to train. So if you make your training sessions either torturous or inconvenient at the start, it won't be long before one of the "good" reasons becomes a "good enough" reason to skip your training. Once that first domino falls, it's hard to reverse the downward trend. Before long, almost any reason becomes a good-enough reason to skip training and then, within days or weeks, you're done. Avoid this ill-fated script by selecting a realistic training time interval and by keeping your initial sessions relatively short and sweet.[7]

Once you've launched into your program and knocked out a few training sessions, you should expect to feel a little soreness, but overall you're going to feel great. The aches and pains will pale in comparison to the overwhelmingly positive sensations produced by accomplishment, success and physical development. If you train smart from the

DEVELOPING A CONSISTENT TRAINING ROUTINE

I often have aspiring and incumbent firefighter/athletes ask me for assistance in developing a personal training program. In an effort to try and help them become consistent in their training, I hand them a four-week calendar (see sample below) and ask them to simply check off each day in which they complete some form of dedicated physical exercise. I tell them that I don't really care what type of exercise they do or quite frankly how long it lasts (even just 5–10 minutes), just as long as it is a truly "dedicated" exercise effort. I always provide a few pointers on training equipment and strongly recommend that they keep their sessions relatively light. In most cases, we also discuss the basic principles of performance-oriented nutrition.

FEBRUARY 2008

Sun	Mon	Tues	Wed	Thurs	Fri	Sat
					1	2
3	4	5	6	7	8	9
10	11	12	13	14	15	16
17	18	19	20	21	22	23
24	25	26	27	28	29	

Exercise: Place a check in the day's box each time you participate in a dedicated exercise session (e.g., walking, running, lifting weights) of at least 5–10 continuous minutes.

Nutrition: Place a plus sign (+) in the day's box for each serving of vegetables, fruits or grains that you eat on the given day. Place one minus (-) in the day's box for each high-fat food item (e.g., fried chicken, french fries, cheese, potato chips, ice cream, chocolate) you eat on that given day.

Then I graciously wish them the best of luck and tell them that I look forward to seeing them again in about a month. Four weeks and 20 or so checks later, they return and we work together to create a sure-fire individualized and progressive training program. The calendar functions as a simplistic training journal, prompting you to complete your daily training sessions and encouraging you to continue to build upon your mounting accomplishments.

Again, the main idea here is to get the firefighter/athletes to prioritize and effectively integrate exercise into their lives. Once they do, they can begin to build a solid base and from there, the sky's the limit. The same naturally applies to you. Once you've developed a consistent training routine, it's no longer a question of if but when your training goals will be achieved. Consistency is the undeniable key to training success.

start and stay consistent with your efforts, you're going to feel great and enjoy continued success.

That's not to say that every training day is going to be a blast. Farther down the road, there will undoubtedly be days when you're less than enthusiastic about your training. Everyone has these days—the door's not locked but you just can't seem to get it opened to get out. On days like these, it's all about taking the first big step. Somehow you have to win the internal argument and get out the door, but how? Easy. Lie to yourself. Tell yourself that you're just going out for a brief jog or a really short circuit. Rationalize that something is always better than nothing when it comes to training and move quickly for the door before you change your mind. Do whatever it takes to close the deal, because once you get out there and start moving, chances are you'll loosen up, snap out of the funk and enjoy a productive session. Even if you don't snap out of it and just wind up completing the short workout, I guarantee that you'll still feel great about the effort. Deep down inside you'll know that, as tough as it was to get out there, you were even tougher. Good triumphed over evil and once again it is confirmed that you *are*, in fact The Man or The Woman!

Once in conversation with a group of FDNY health and fitness instructors on the topic of firefighter candidate physical ability testing, one instructor suggested that "the best physical assessment for hire would be a candidate's performance in the New York City Marathon."[1] On the surface this may seem as excessive and invalid to you now as it did to the rest of us sitting around the table at the time; however, it actually made an interesting point. Acknowledging that firefighters must be physically well conditioned to safely and effectively perform their job, it then follows that firefighters must train consistently in order to maintain the necessary level of physical fitness. What better tool to measure a person's commitment to consistent training than the local running event in which individuals can only achieve success as a result of consistent training? Naturally, firefighters need to be much more than just aerobically fit to get the job done. The point we make again with the use of this example is that your success in training, just like that of all firefighter/athletes, depends to the greatest extent upon your being able to train consistently.

STEP 4. Build Gradual, Intelligent Progressions

Most people fail in self-initiated training efforts because they set their initial training goals much too high. They wind up doing too much too soon, and then drop out as a consequence of frustration, undue discomfort or injury. In the words of FDNY Fire Marshal (retired) Mike Andreachi, "They blast off and burn out like nickel rockets." Why? Because with the best of intentions and great enthusiasm they bite off much more than they can chew. They create workouts for themselves that are too long, too difficult and too painful. This negative experience results in a subconscious desire to quit. The desire grows quickly, and, before long, they quit. Don't make this same fatal mistake: Design your program to succeed; start out nice and easy. Remember, when it comes to beginning a new program, "light is right" and, very often, "less is more."

The roles of psychology and psychological perspective in training cannot be denied. In order to succeed in your training, you have to stay motivated, and in order to stay motivated you need some form of consistent positive feedback. Consistent positive feedback can be obtained through steady achievement. This is best accomplished through the completion of a well-designed, progressive series of realistic short-term goals.

To successfully build upon your initial gains, you should gradually increase the frequency (number of sessions each week) of your workouts, progressively building to the point where you're training aerobically nearly every day and/or strength training three or four times a week. The second progressive adjustment that you should consider making would be to increase the duration (length, time or distance of sessions) of your workouts. Finally, after developing a sound training foundation, you should consider elevating the intensity (how hard you train) of your sessions.

Progressively increasing your training challenges with the intent to inspire positive development is referred to as the "overload principle of training." In the beginning, only minor increases in training frequency, duration or intensity are recommended, just enough to slightly overload the targeted muscles, tissues and systems. Mild to moderate levels of training overload will encourage the development of desirable changes. However, if you train too hard, the overload stimulus is likely to cause significant tissue damage and injury. Remember, in the long run, small progressive steps accomplish the most significant gains. As you continue with your program you should closely monitor your progress and, when appropriate, make progressive adjustments in response to improvement. Just be careful not to overdo it. This is the most common mistake in training, one which too often results in pain, injury, disgust and failure.

In the fire service, it's acknowledged that if you take big steps on a smoky roof, you are likely to take a fatal fall. The same holds true of physical training. Start out conservatively and then build slowly and progressively through time. Establish a series of meaningful and graduated short-term goals and then just slowly and steadily ascend the training ladder of success. In using this intelligent approach to training, you'll be much more likely to maintain a higher level of motivation, minimize your risk of training-related injury and experience continued success. Small progressive steps ultimately lead to the largest gains.

STEP 5. Balanced Training

The human body is an amazing bio-machine, miraculously responding to vigorous challenges by improving its ability to better handle them in the future. Think about it: You exercise a muscle to the point of exhaustion, and the body's automatic response is to increase that muscle's ability to better resist fatigue. It's an incredible feature to possess; all you have to do is support it by eating the right foods, staying well hydrated and getting sufficient rest.

Maintaining a proper balance between exercise and rest is crucial to producing rapid and significant gains. The key is to maintain the balance. Sometimes this is easy but other times it's not, particularly at the onset of a program when your motivation is at its peak, or a little further down the road where dramatic early gains provide abundant positive feedback. Be careful not to over do it in the beginning, and try not to get carried away with yourself as a result of early successes.

Once you've been training for a while, you'll likely notice some very desirable improvements and naturally want to develop even more. The question then becomes, "How do you continue to ride the crest of this positive training wave without either falling back and plateauing or pushing too hard and crashing over the other side?" In other words, how do you script your training program to develop a balance that produces optimal development and continued gains?

One safe and productive way to maintain proper balance in your progressive training is to employ a "hard–easy" approach. Alternate the intensity and duration of your training so that you never train either "hard" or "long" two days in a row. By insuring a day's rest between training sessions or, for more experienced athletes, by either completing a lighter session of training between harder workouts or alternating body areas with lifting, the body is provided sufficient time to rebuild, re-fuel and otherwise improve itself. As the body adapts and develops, you can gradually increase the intensity, duration and frequency of your training. This is the sure-fire path to training success. Of note, however, is that with increased age you may find (as we have) that you'll enjoy greater success employing a "hard–easy–easy" approach. For reasons not yet clearly defined, the body's ability to recuperate and develop (among other things) slows as we age.

WARNING: If you do not supply your body with the appropriate nutrients and/or allow adequate time for recovery with your training, the exercise stress that could and should have been *constructive* winds up instead being absolutely *destructive*. Your imbalanced overtraining will produce lethargy and chronic fatigue, and injury to muscle, tendon, ligament and skeletal tissue are likely to result.

Another important aspect of balanced training involves the principle of balanced muscular development. Back injury is the most common debilitating injury suffered by working firefighters. It's also a major problem for many middle-aged Americans, especially those who are de-conditioned and overfat. A number of different factors may be responsible for promoting the occurrence of this type of injury on the job. One factor is muscular imbalance: the disproportionate development (overdevelopment vs. underdevelopment) of muscles in different areas of the body. If you picture your body as a skeleton encased by a series of interconnected and overlapping muscles, you can see that the muscular system functions in a manner similar to a chain. To enable movement and the execution of physical tasks, muscles must work in a coordinated and therefore codependent manner. Therefore, as you swing powerfully to force open a steel door

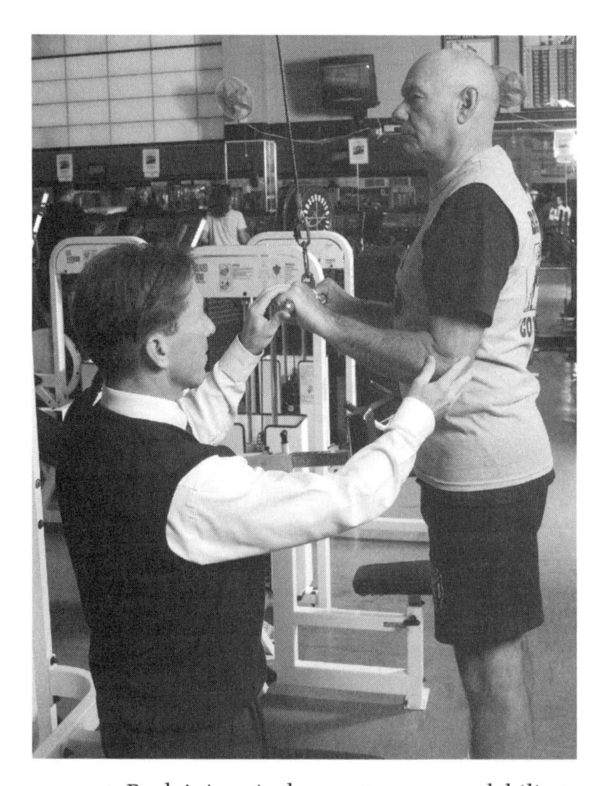

with your maul, or as you rotate your trunk to avoid a defensive player on the basketball court, you involve several major muscle groups and place significant demands on nearly every link of the chain. If every muscle in the chain is sufficiently conditioned and therefore fit enough to contend with the imposed demand, your performance is successful and no injury results. However, if one muscle or muscle group is significantly less conditioned (weaker) than the others involved, it, as the weak link in the chain, is the most likely to become injured. This commonly occurs with the lower back, as people tend to focus more on the development of other body areas: the chest, shoulders, arms, abdominals and legs. The easiest way to avoid this common pitfall is by utilizing a total-body resistance-training program. If you already participate in some form of resistance training, take a look at your current program and make certain that you're hitting all areas of the body. Be careful—"don't fall in love with your favorite exercise."[12] Keep your training comprehensive and well balanced to ensure proper total-body development.

STEP 6. Get Yourself Checked Out

Before launching into a rigorous training routine, you need to be certain that your body is absolutely ready to contend with the intense demands. Getting yourself checked out by a physician prior to beginning a new program is therefore an excellent idea. Many medical conditions such as heart disease and high blood pressure can develop without producing any noticeable symptoms and therefore exist without you ever becoming aware. For this reason, they are referred to as "silent killers." "You don't want the joker popping up in the deck."[1] Suffering a preventable heart attack is the exact opposite of what you're trying to achieve. Have your physician minimize that ill-fated potential prior to the onset of your training.

Firefighters should receive a comprehensive medical/physical exam prior to employment, and then annually throughout the term of their careers. Your approach should be the same. Get yourself checked out by a physician prior to launching into a new physical training program, especially if you've already celebrated your 40th birthday. Again, using the analogy of preparing for a family trip: the older the car, the more important a thorough inspection before the ride.

In this regard, I had a good friend a few years back who was an outstanding firefighter in one of the busiest fire companies on the job. He had been out of the field for a while on an off-line assignment and was significantly de-conditioned as a result. Like so many other great firefighters, he decided one day to get back in shape. Believing himself to be healthy and tough enough to handle the physical and physiological demands of his training, he charged right into his training with the same fearlessness and aggressiveness he was known for in the field. He didn't have himself medically cleared first and tragedy resulted. Make sure you're ready to go *before* you begin your training.

STEP 7. Conduct Assessments

Once you're medically cleared and ready to begin training, you need to determine the current abilities of the specific muscles and related body systems that you wish to develop. You can achieve this by conducting basic pre-test measures of the fitness element(s) and parameter(s) you wish to improve. In the FDNY academy, we achieved this through the use of fundamental fitness tests like the 1.5-

mile run, bent-knee sit-ups, push-ups and reverse-grip pull-ups. You can easily conduct your own personal aerobic fitness test by running, cycling or swimming in whatever venue or environment you intend to train: the track, road or local pool. The same goes for resistance training. Just head on down to your basement or the gym in which you intend to train and measure your initial ability to perform each exercise of your workout routine.

To ensure the highest degree of validity with your exercise testing, you should enter the session appropriately dressed, well rested, properly fueled and sufficiently hydrated. If you are resistance training in an organized gym, always map out your exercise series before the onset of your session. This way you'll know in advance where to go when moving from one exercise to the next. Also, it's a good idea to locate back-up stations as alternates in case your primary station (piece of equipment) is in use when you arrive. You don't want to get stuck standing around waiting for someone to complete multiple sets. This will cause you to lose focus and cool down, both of which are counterproductive. Also, be certain to stretch and warm up prior to the testing session and cool down immediately afterwards. These actions will improve test performance, minimize the risk of injury and facilitate recovery. Finally, we recommend that you proceed in a safe and conservative manner. If you're completing a resistance training circuit, move directly from one exercise to the next, but take the time during each exercise to move smoothly and "mindfully"[12] through the full range of motion, maintaining excellent form at all times. If you're involved with aerobic testing, avoid the common error of going out too fast and fizzling out. This will produce an unpleasant experience and inaccurate results. Move smart and then tough; hold back a little at the onset and proceed at a more moderate intensity, then slowly and progressively build to a strong crescendo at the finish.

There are many different formulas that you can use to calculate the appropriate starting weights for the exercises of your personal training routine. In general, they're based upon the amount of weight that you can successfully move in one or a few repetitions with maximal effort. However, in keeping with our general philosophy of "simple is good," we suggest that you pre-test yourself by running through the personalized training set you developed as it was designed. Complete the exercises in their pre-scripted order and record the weight that you're able to successfully move through the full range of motion for at least the minimum number

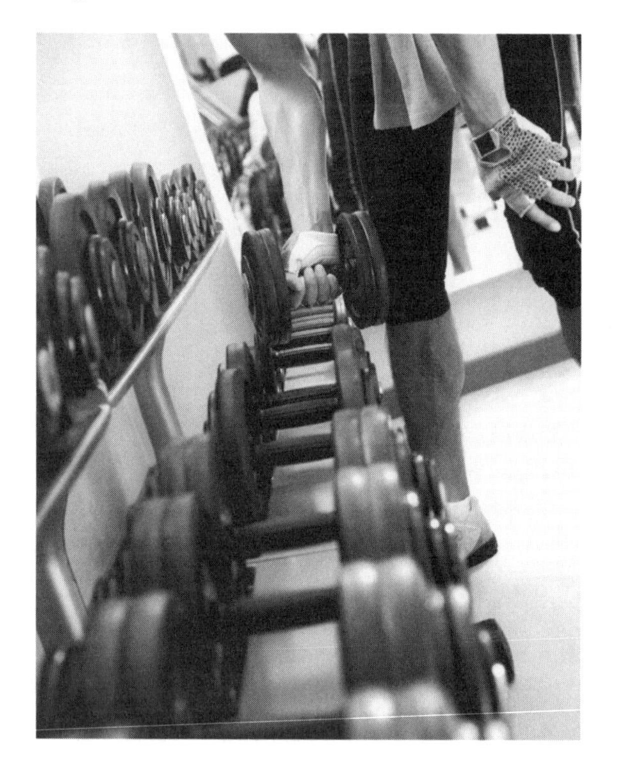

of prescribed repetitions. As an example, if the number of repetitions that you plan to complete for a given exercise is 15–20, then the selected pre-test weight should be one in which you're able to complete at least 15 times and not more than 20 (without breaking form or experiencing undue strain).

Again, when selecting the appropriate weights for resistance training, you're far better off starting out a little light than too heavy. If you push too hard at the onset, excessive discomfort, frustration and injury are likely to result. On the other hand, if you start out a little bit more conservatively, you'll enjoy greater initial gains and a more positive training experience. This is the formula for success. The same basic truths apply to aerobic training, where the pre-test based selection of training distance or duration, and intensity should be conservatively applied to enhance the prospect of training enjoyment, improvement and success.

STEP 8. Use Appropriate Equipment

When selecting the proper clothing and equipment for your training, there's no better rule of thumb to apply than simply using the right tool for the job. Training attire and equipment should be chosen on the basis of their abilities to facilitate training gains and performance. The type of activity, session intensity and duration, level of ability and weather all play a role in determining what clothing is best to wear and what equipment is best to use. Just give it some thought and try to use what is safest and most productive rather than what just happens to be handy or is the least expensive. You don't have to spend a fortune to acquire good clothing and equipment, but if you go for the low-end product, there's a good chance that you'll get precisely what you paid for. If you get injured as a result of using inexpensive poor-quality clothing and equipment, then all of a sudden, "cheap becomes expensive."

Clothing

For the most part, deciding what to wear for a workout is only as complicated as you make it. Selecting performance-oriented attire is simple; it's only "fashion" that complicates the matter. If you keep in mind that you're dressing for a workout rather than a date, then aside from the state of your sneakers, suiting up for a session should be an effortless task.

Clothing design varies as a function of training activity and environment; however, some basic principles universally apply. Loose-fitting shirts and pants (or shorts) allow for greater freedom of movement and facilitate body cooling. It's clearly beneficial to be unencumbered as you move quickly and dynamically, and the accumulation of excessive body heat is something that needs to be avoided. Cotton items designed for activity, especially socks and shirts, are a good low-cost choice, given their ability to breathe and wick perspiration from the skin. Slick materials may also be useful in the prevention of chafing between the legs, chest and arms.

Wearing clothing that will keep your body warm as you move through a resistance-training circuit may be productive, especially in a cooler gym; however, don't wear clothing that inhibits free movement, overinsulates or traps sweat. In short, "warm is good, but hot is not." In cool windy weather, wearing a wind-resistant outer shell of clothing, along with gloves and a cap, helps to preserve body heat. This is key in preventing illness related to low body temperature and injury to the fingers and ears. When exercising at high intensities or in hot,

SPECIAL CONSIDERATIONS FOR WOMEN

Historically, athletics and sport have been a breeding ground for flawed assumptions in terms of a woman's athletic abilities, training development potentials and capacities. Misinformation, as well as the absence of legitimate information about female physical and physiological development have slowed the ability of female athletes to reach their full potentials and ascend to elite levels. As a prime example, it wasn't until 1984 that the women's marathon became an Olympic event. Recent advances in training and a greater understanding of the female physiology have, however, allowed women of all ages to become more prominent in physically demanding professions and athletics. The following is some important information relevant to the specialized needs and training considerations for women firefighter/athletes.

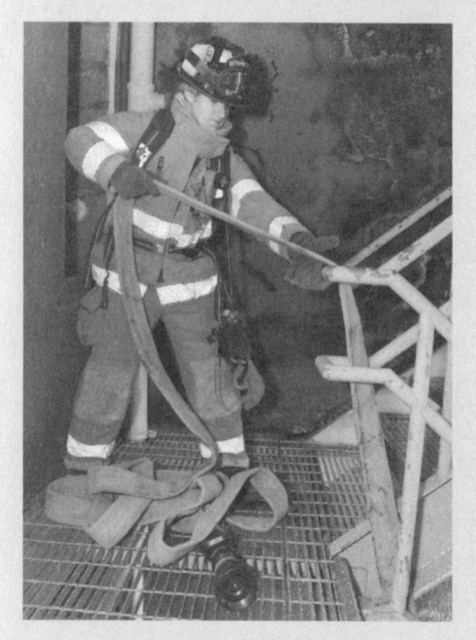

Aerobic Training: On the average, women have an aerobic capacity that is 7–10 percent lower than that of men. This is primarily due to the fact that women have approximately 10 percent lower hemoglobin content in their blood.[9] Importantly, women appear to adapt to aerobic training in a manner quite similar to men, except that the more prominent changes occur within the muscle, resulting in the enhancement of muscle cell ability to take up and utilize oxygen to produce energy. Women runners who have broad hips are likely to experience greater stress on the musculoskeletal components of their hips, knees and ankles. To minimize the potential for injury, good-quality sneakers and a commitment to stretching are a must. Working a comprehensive resistance-training circuit to improve total-body muscular endurance would also be beneficial.

Strength Training: In general, men feature a greater ability to develop muscle size, strength and power than women. This results from the production of larger amounts of the muscle-building hormone testosterone. What is critically important to understand, however, is that women still possess the same quality of

humid weather, and when performing aerobic exercises that involve a large muscle mass like running, stair stepping and riding a stationary cycle, it's best to wear clothing that allows air, vaporized sweat and water to escape; this helps cool the body and prevent overheating.

WARNING: Wearing a nylon or rubber suit when exercising intensely in a warm environment is a misguided and extremely dangerous act. The dehydration and increase in core body temperature that result can cause serious injury. Moreover, exercise capacity is dramatically reduced and nearly all of the noted weight loss is due to accelerated dehydration. Therefore, in wearing these ridiculous outfits, not only do you adversely impact your training efforts, you also place yourself at risk of injury and the water weight you lose is almost immediately regained.

Some people find hand equipment like lifting grips or gloves to be useful, especially when training with dumbbells, barbells and heavier weights.

muscle fiber and that they can therefore develop tremendous muscular endurance, strength and power with proper training. Additionally, women generally feature a lower center of gravity and a broader natural base of support, both of which aid in providing a more stable base of support for the execution of resistance-training exercises in a standing position.

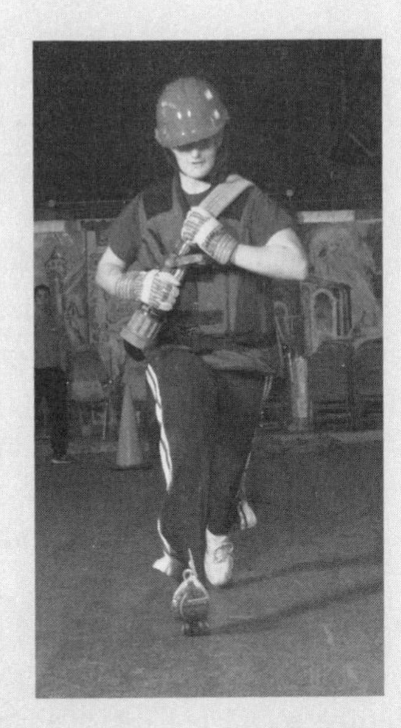

Flexibility Training: Women who frequently wear shoes with elevated heels are likely to develop a shortening of the muscle-tendon complex in the calf region (gastrocnemius and soleus muscles, and Achilles tendon) of the lower hind leg. To avoid tendon sprains and muscle strains caused by the dramatic stretching of the shortened tissue when exercising in sneakers, considerable attention should be paid to thoroughly stretching this muscle-tendon region before and after each training session.

Body Cooling: Women have a very efficient body-cooling system that enables them to cool themselves without losing nearly as much body water via sweat as men. Proper hydration is still a critical issue, though, and special consideration must be given to the performance of high-intensity work or exercise in hot and humid weather.

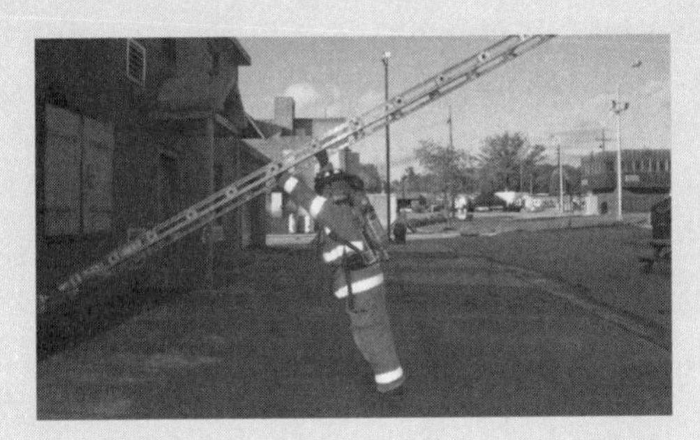

Nutrition: Akin to men, women require specific nutrients to train hard and perform at their highest level. It particular, it has been noted that women should make a conscientious effort to consume foods that provide them with sufficient amounts of iron to support the production of oxygen-carrying hemoglobin and red blood cells, calcium to enable muscle contraction, phosphorus to work together with calcium to build strong bones, and magnesium to ensure bone health and facilitate energy metabolism.

Having a solid and secure grip improves lifting safety and execution. Finally, for reasons of personal hygiene, comfort and safety, it's always a good idea to bring along a hand towel to wipe the equipment cushions before and after you exercise.

In terms of obtaining proper footwear, the simple truth is that what's good for the goose may not be good for the gander. Given that the foot shape, foot strike, running gait, body mass and training demands are different with each unique individual, it's easy to understand why no one sneaker fits all. As an example, one year, ten FDNY members ran the New York City Marathon in under three hours, each wearing a different model of sneaker. Different types and brands of sneakers have different designs and therefore feature a different fit. Thus, the best sneaker for *you* is the one that fits you most comfortably and meets your particular training needs.

In general, your training shoes and sneakers should be stable and provide good arch support.

For high-impact exercises like running, greater shock absorption is also important. However, in other forms of activity like basketball, where stability is a major issue, a lower heel may provide a better base of support. Given the importance of obtaining proper footwear with running, beginning runners should consider seeking out a knowledgeable salesperson in a specialized runner's shop to make sure that the shoe they get fits right and meets their specific training needs. In New York City, at any one of the many Super Runners shops, you can get this level of service and (with permission) actually take a few strides outside. Owner Gary Murche is a retired NYC firefighter and the winner of the first NYC Marathon. His sales staff is largely composed of experienced and successful runners so you're likely to obtain the shoes that fit you best in all regards.

Equipment

The low cost, versatility and exceptional health benefits of running make it an outstanding training choice. For the price of a pair of sneakers, you can train in virtually any type of weather, anytime and anywhere. Treadmill training is a convenient option at times, especially in bad weather. Just be conscious of the fact that when training aerobically indoors, you're likely to lose quite a bit of body fluid via sweat due to the lack of ventilation. Therefore, you'll need to drink more hydrating fluids before and after each session. One more word on treadmills: Be careful not to overdo it with the elevation feature. A little bit of work at increased elevation is fine, but too much can place undue stress on your feet, ankles, hips, knees and lower back.

Most of the aerobic equipment provided in organized gyms is of sufficient quality to provide

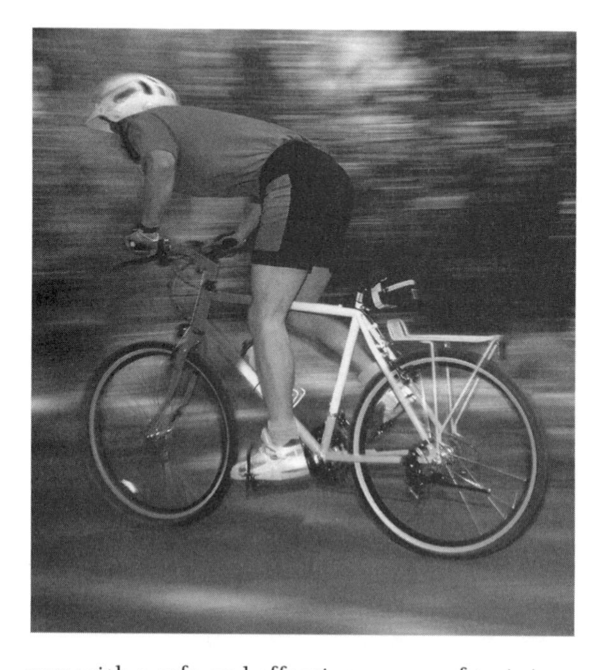

you with a safe and effective means of training. Some pieces of equipment, like the cross-country skiing machine, may require a little more effort to master, but most are very easy to use. Your real challenge then is to decide which type of exercise is best for you. If you want to focus more on just your legs, then cycling, stair climbing and running are the way to go. On the other hand, if you want to simultaneously develop your trunk and arms, then you might want to give either rowing or cross-country skiing a try. All of these tools provide excellent training stimuli and can therefore produce outstanding training effects.

The wide variety of weight-training equipment that exists in most gyms makes the development of a resistance-training program fairly easy. If you're planning to train in a less formal setting such as your home, you may wish to keep things simple. An excellent total body workout can be achieved with just the use of lightweight dumbbells and calisthenics exercises. That's how we trained the FDNY Academy probationary firefighters. With the use of a small mat for protection from the asphalt surface and two 20-pound dumbbells, we worked through a full spectrum of exercises and completed a variety of challenging total body workouts. You can do the same. The other option, of course, is to create a more elaborate home gym. We recommend that you use good-quality equipment and keep things simple at the start. Calisthenics and free-weight versions of all of our resistance training programs are provided in the upcoming chapter on strength training (page 65).

For individuals with little or no previous weight-training experience, resistance machines are a very safe, uncomplicated and efficient way to begin. You can very easily pick through the broad selection of machines offered in most gyms to develop an effective total-body training circuit. Resistance machines assist with the coordination of movement. Illustrated instructions are often attached to the side of the machine, but if not, instructors are usually available to provide guidance. As you proceed through your circuit, concentrate on developing good form and lifting techniques so that you can ultimately progress to the use of free weights.

For experienced lifters, cable systems, barbells and dumbbells are often the preferred choice. Here you can vary the plane of motion to match and thereby improve the ability of muscles involved in almost any desired movement. Motor skills are keenly developed and the capacities of supporting muscles are greatly enhanced. The completion of strenuous firefighting tasks involves a variety of movements through many different planes of motion, not offered through the use of most resistance machines. Consequently, progressing to the predominant use of cable machines and free weights would be most productive for high-performance athletes as well as active and aspiring firefighters.

SAMPLE JOURNAL PAGE

Sunday 3/17/08

Sunny, windy, 46°F

175 lbs

DIET

Breakfast: A large bowl of raisin bran with skim milk & a cup of coffee.

Lunch: A bowl of vegetable soup, buttered bagel, blueberry muffin & a cup of coffee.

Dinner: Roast beef, green beans, and mashed potatoes with gravy.

Snacks: Small bag of pretzels & a piece of cake.

EXERCISE

Workout: 10 minutes of stretching. 5 minutes of jogging, two full circuits of weights and 5 more minutes of jogging. 10 minutes of light stretching.

Training Journal

Training progress is easy to measure and define when you keep an accurate record of sessions, sets, exercises and repetitions, thus we highly recommend that you use a training journal to record and review all of your training activities. In keeping a daily training journal, you'll compose a permanent record of your training history, progress and achievements. This will assist you in developing a better understanding of your individual training and performance potentials and abilities. In athletics, the training journal is often referred to as "the book of truths"[3] because a well-kept journal provides the honest answer to almost any question about your training progress or performance. There are few mysteries or surprises in athletic performance or training when an athlete maintains an accurate training journal. Another good reason for maintaining a journal is that the written evidence of your training efforts serves as a great source of inspiration and motivation. Just like reviewing the pages of a savings account booklet, you're going to feel great and become motivated to do even more as you review the progress which results from your consistent training (deposits).

You can get as complicated as you'd like with your journal entries; however, we recommend that you keep things simple so that they're easy to do

TRAINING SESSION CHART

NAME: David Spierer DATE: 2/23
HRpre: 70 HRpost: 132 Time: 32:00

EXERCISE	LBS	REPS	LBS	REPS
Leg Press	176	20	176	20
Seated Chest	110	20	110	18
Vert Butterfly	60	20	60	19
Shoulder Press	40	20	40	20
Lat Pull–Curl	90	20	90	20
Triceps Extension	40	20	40	17
Seated Row	85	20	85	20
Calf Raise	170	20	170	20
Leg Extension	70	20	70	17
Leg Curl	70	20	70	19
Abdominal	100	20	100	20
Lower Back	150	20	150	20

NOTES: Increase shoulder press, 40 to 45

and therefore more likely to get done. List the form (e.g., aerobic or strength) and/or specific type of exercise (e.g., running or circuit training), and then draft a brief description of your workout. For aerobic athletes, it's important to include a description of exercise intensity and duration, running terrain and the weather (for example: Ran 5 miles in 37:40, hilly course, cool and windy). With resistance training, it is helpful to record more detailed information. You may therefore want to complete a more extensive training session chart (see page 26). Resistance-training session charts are easy to develop and simple to use. If you belong to a gym, chances are they already have blank charts printed up and ready to use.

Provided on page 26 is an example of the type of training chart our firefighter/athletes use in recording their resistance (weight) training session efforts. The chart is placed on a clipboard and filled out as the athlete progresses through the workout. After completing the training session, the athlete files the chart in his/her personal training binder. Keeping accurate daily records like this enables you to monitor your progress and make proper decisions when considering program changes. It increases both the efficiency and effectiveness of your training. Measuring your heart rate prior to and immediately after training and recording the amount of time it takes for you to complete your training session provides you with some productive feedback relevant to the intensity of the day's session.

There are some additional journal entries that you may want to make in order to provide a more definitive history of your efforts and progress. For instance, it's always a good idea to evaluate your relative state of hydration by measuring and recording your daily weight. You may also want to provide a brief description of your diet. Although this may seem tedious at times, it's often quite revealing and therefore very productive with training programs designed to lose body weight (fat). If done consistently, a comprehensive training journal can provide you with invaluable feedback, motivation and insight relative to your personal training gains and potentials.

Pictured on page 25 is a sample journal page that includes descriptions of both diet and physical training. If you're purely interested in recording your training activity, the entries are extremely short and may actually be filled in on a standard calendar.

Nutrition

The effect of sound nutrition on physical performance, appearance and health are undeniable. Simply stated, if you want to look, feel and move like a Ferrari, you'd better consume a diet rich in high-octane foods. And if you choose to eat like a hog, don't expect to move like a gazelle. Nutrition is a critical piece of the training puzzle. What you eat is clearly going to either boost or hinder your physical development and performance. Give this a thought—the next time you walk past a fast-food restaurant, look through the window and observe the consequences of adverse consumption. Is that where you want to be? Probably not, especially if you're reading this book. You want to look great, feel great and perform at the highest level. You want to be "firefighter fit," and to achieve this goal you need to learn how to become a mindful consumer—eating right, often and light. You need to consume a performance-oriented diet rich in "foods that fuel you up and clean you out rather than those that slow you down and clog you up."[12] And as you do, you'll undoubtedly see how the human body, when properly nourished, can do amazing things.

This chapter provides you with the information you need to develop an important understanding of healthful and performance-oriented nutrition. Our approach to performance nutrition is simple, proven, realistic and effective. You'll find it easy to understand and simple to apply. In learning the basic facts and principles we put forth in the following pages, you'll be able to create your own personalized high-performance diet—a diet that fits your particular tastes and promotes optimal training development and performance.

Simple Truth #1: Your mother was right.

It's always nice to begin a new section on a positive note. That said, the good news here is that the diverse, well-balanced and complex carbohydrate-based diet that your mother provided and insisted that you eat was right on the mark. She knew of your tremendous potential early on and therefore fueled you to achieve great success from the start. Her emphasis on whole foods; cereals, fruits and vegetables was sheer genius. She was your first great coach, but now it's time for you to take over the helm and surge ahead.

In line with your mother's intuitive prescription, we recommend that you consume a diet composed of approximately 55 to 60 percent carbohydrate (primarily complex starches, *not* simple sugars), about 15 percent protein, and less than 30 percent fat. Moreover, you should absolutely minimize your saturated fat intake (less than 10 percent) and avoid trans fatty acids at all costs. Fluid intake should include the bountiful consumption of caffeine- and alcohol-free beverages. If your diet is well balanced (as described) and truly diverse in terms of selected food items, then supplementation with any form of chemical (vitamin, mineral, predigested amino acids, magical herbs) is unwarranted. Having said that, if you wish to augment your nutritional intake with a basic multi-vitamin/multi-mineral for the sake of personal assurance or insurance, go right ahead, "no harm, no foul."[11]

If you maintain this balance (55 to 60 percent carbohydrate/roughly 15 percent protein/less than 30 percent fat) and diversify your food item selection, you'll obtain adequate amounts of all the nutrients (including protein) necessary to train and develop optimally. We caution you *not* to fall prey to the slick and seductive marketing efforts of the billion-dollar supplement industry. Consuming the questionable contents from a tremendous jar of "Nitro-muscle Super Blaster" (or whatever) most certainly will *not* result in the miraculous development of monster-sized muscles like those of air-brushed Nitro-man, nor will it land you a date with his counterpart Nitro-woman. Eating smart and training intelligently are the ways to get you to where you want to go—*not* some magic potion, powder or pill.

Further emphasizing the importance of diversifying the food items on your personal menu, we make the point that falling in love with your favorite food or consuming a "one-food wonder" diet is as unhealthy as it is unproductive. In both cases, the resulting diets are nutritionally flawed, as no one food provides the broad range of nutrients necessary to meet all of your physiologic needs. Diversity is the key to nutritional success. Make a concerted effort to select and consume a variety of different types of foods, emphasizing fruits, vegetables and whole-grain choices. This will enable you to obtain the full spectrum of nutrients necessary to promote good health and high-quality performance.

Simple Truth #2: Carbohydrate is the fuel for the fire floor.

Carbohydrate is the primary source of fuel for firefighting and the performance of other high-intensity physical activities. It's also the preferred source of fuel for muscles performing moderate to high-intensity aerobic work, red blood cells delivering oxygen to working muscles, and brain cells that enable you to think. Unlike protein and fat, this is the fuel that facilitates high-level mental and physical performance in critical and demanding situations. Thus, to perform on the level of a high-intensity firefighter or high-performance athlete, you need to consume a carbohydrate-based high-performance diet.

McArdle,[9] Pritiken,[13] Bailey[2] and a league of other similarly knowledgeable nutritionists all recommend that carbohydrate make up the majority of your daily caloric intake. We agree, and for one good reason: It works! However, recognizing that percentages are often difficult to calculate though the course of a day, we suggest that you initially employ the following simple fix: Substitute high-quality complex carbohydrate foods (fruits, vegetables, cereals, juices and whole-grain products) for some of the lower-quality fatty foods that you might otherwise be inclined to devour. In so doing, not only will you be loading up your body with the high-performance fuel it requires and desires, but you'll also be supplying it with the essential vitamins, minerals, fiber and water it needs to promote good health and powerhouse performance. The more you move in the direction of whole-food consumption, the sooner you'll realize the incredible truth that you can actually *eat more and weigh less.*[5]

Simple Truth #3: Eat foods that fuel you up and clean you out.

This simple truth also emphasizes carbohydrate intake since the consumption of complex-carbohydrate foods support high-end physical performance, and assists in the prevention of both heart

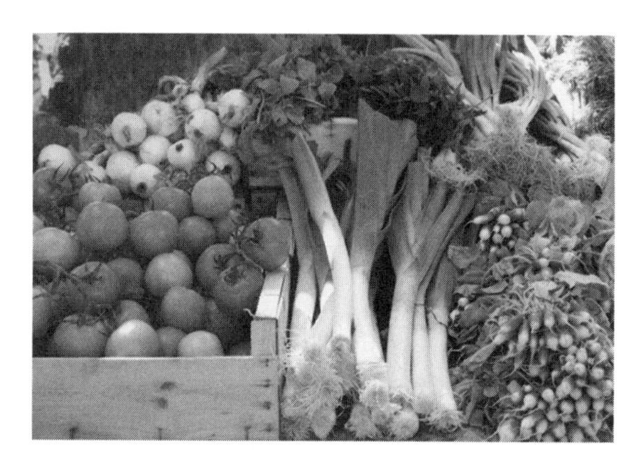

disease and cancer. A diet rich in (complex) carbohydrates such as fruits, vegetables, cereals, grains, juices, rice and pasta provides you with the fuel you need to perform at your highest level. Fat, on the other hand, will only contribute significantly as a source of fuel during the performance of low- to moderate-intensity aerobic exercise, and protein has to be scavenged from body tissue and then converted to carbohydrate in the liver before it's used as a viable energy source. Consequently, diets that are high in protein and fat rather than carbohydrate are likely to fill you up with unusable fuels and simultaneously starve you of the "rocket" fuel you need to perform—a diet high in protein and fat will cause you to fatigue more rapidly as unfilled muscle and liver stores of carbohydrate quickly deplete. This will have an undeniably negative effect on both your training and athletic or firefighting performance.

WARNING: High-protein diets are particularly dangerous to high-performance firefighter/athletes. They fail to provide adequate carbohydrate fuel and promote the loss of essential body water, electrolyte minerals and the water-soluble vitamins used for producing energy. Dehydration can accelerate the rate of fatigue and diminish the body's ability for cooling during high-intensity physical work or exercise, especially in hot and humid athletic, training and firefighting environments. Thus, consuming a high-protein, low-carbohydrate diet that results in carbohydrate depletion and dehydration is unproductive, unhealthy and potentially lethal for high-intensity firefighter/athletes.

If you consume our recommended performance diet, not only will you likely improve your mental and physical performances, you'll also be offering your body added protection from developing heart disease and cancer, the number one and two killers of Americans. Firefighters in particular are susceptible to the development of certain forms of cancer because of their exposure to toxins. Heart disease is also a major issue; heart attacks often claim the lives of more working firefighters than all other causes of death combined. To limit the possibilities of developing atherosclerosis (hardening of the arteries) or high blood pressure and suffering a heart attack or stroke, you need to minimize your intake of cholesterol containing animal flesh, whole-fat dairy products and fried foods. Simultaneously, you should increase your consumption of nutritious whole foods containing soluble and insoluble forms of fiber.

Soluble fiber binds to cholesterol-rich bile in your intestine and drags it out the southern end. This elegant action can significantly reduce the body's total cholesterol, a leading risk factor for the development of heart disease. Insoluble fiber seems to help reduce the potential for developing certain forms of cancer, including colorectal cancer; a particular hazard for firefighters. To understand the protective actions of insoluble fiber, think of broccoli. The non-digestible, insoluble flowerets and stalk act as nature's scrub brush, wiping undesirable and potentially lethal (pre-cancerous) products from the intestinal walls as they move through the digestive tract. The easiest way to increase your fiber intake is to eat more sensationally nutritious whole foods: fruits, vegetables, cereals and grains (seven to nine servings, according to Dr. Charles Bens, nutritionist and noted author).

The most popular human in the firehouse most mornings is the one who enters the kitchen with a bag of donuts. These sugar-coated, trans fatty acid–fried rings of processed flour represent the pinnacle of anti-performance nutrition; however, there's no denying that they're delicious, especially with a fresh cup of firehouse brew. So how do you deal with this internal conflict? Do you try and cut back a little on the donuts, or do you just completely cut them out cold turkey? Read ahead for the answer.

Simple Truth #4: Moderation is the key.

Good news on the donut front—just cut back! Research has shown that moderate consumption rather than forced abstention is clearly the way to go. Hey, who knows, maybe you're the kind of super-human that can just cut the stinkin' donuts out. Don't count on it, though, because with most normal humans this approach just doesn't work. When people deny themselves of something they really enjoy, like a greasy, frosted donut, they typically win the internal battle of denial for a few days, but then for whatever reason cave in and consume half the box. Diets of denial just don't work! The more successful strategy seems to be to gain a nutritional education that will enable you to become a more mindful consumer, learning to distinguish between good, bad and ugly foods. Then apply what you've learned by consuming more of the recognized high-quality foods while still enjoying (in moderation) the lesser-quality delights. Fill up on the good stuff and, remember, when it comes to the consumption of your favorite foul foods, *moderation is the key to success.*

Simple Truth #5: If you take in more than you put out, you get fat.

We realize this is one of the more obvious truths, one that may encourage you to skip or scan the words ahead. However, we urge you to hang in there for some critical and surprising details. It's important for all firefighter/athletes to understand the concept of energy balance: the relationship between diet, physical exercise or work and body fat loss or gain. The basic equation goes something like this: if you take in more food energy than you or expend, the excess energy accumulates and gets stored as body fat. That's the part you probably already know. Now for the more interesting stuff.

If you take in too much of any kind of fat, be it good fat (unsaturated), bad fat (saturated) or ugly fat (trans fatty acids), your body very simply modifies it and then stores it as body fat. That's pretty straightforward. Less straightforward and clearly less well-known is that if you take in too much protein, most of that beyond what you immediately use is also converted into and stored as body fat. I know this is a particularly painful thought for the protein-shake-and-raw-egg-in-the-morning kinda guy, but it *is* a physiological fact. The excess amino acids that you take in with the consumption of a high-priced protein shake do *not* get stored in some convenient amino acid reservoir nor are they miraculously employed to build additional muscle tissue.

Rather, they are largely converted into and stored as body fat. Carbohydrate follows a similarly tragic biochemical script. Whether you over-consume simple or complex carbohydrates, all of that beyond what you immediately use or store in either muscle tissue or the liver, is converted into and stored as body fat.

Who would have thought that the over-consumption of carbohydrate or protein would be so similar to eating a stick of butter? Well, cholesterol aside, it most certainly is. That's why people who eat a lot of carbohydrate get fat. It's not so much the type of food (carbohydrate) that they're eating as it is the excessive quantity they ingest. It tastes good and it goes down easy. There's plenty of sumptuous carbs on the platter so you keep wolfing them down; they digest rapidly and move into your body fast. They quickly flood your bloodstream, saturate the muscles and then even top off your liver stores. Unfortunately, the remaining excess carbs are then tragically converted into and stored as body fat.

Trained athletes can dramatically increase their capacity to store carbohydrate as glycogen within muscle tissue. This is a definite plus, but you can only store so much. Consequently, if you suck down a humongous bowl of spaghetti at the pre-race pasta party, not only are you carbo-loading but you're also quite paradoxically lard-loading. How much sense does that make when you're going out to run a marathon the next day?

Among those who work and/or train hard, or are frequently confronted with extreme danger and death, there seems a pronounced desire to celebrate life. As such, in the firehouse we had a tendency to regard every day as a holiday and every meal as a feast.[4] This festive philosophy, combined with the belief that "if you work hard, you have got to eat big,"[4] likely inspired the common practice of using platters as opposed to plates in the fire service. Large plates, of course, inspire large meals, and big meals encourage overeating. Additionally, if you were conditioned as a child to eat everything on your plate, then the chances are even greater that whatever sits on the plate before you is going to find its way into your mouth. Solution: Try serving dinner on dessert plates. Only kidding—regular human-sized plates will do the trick. A smaller plate equals less food, less consumption and a happier, healthier life. It's that simple, unless you're the type who's inclined to make additional trips to the stove. That being the case, all bets are off. (P.S. Multi-trip folks may benefit from reading this section more than once.)

Two other factors that promote over-consumption are fast and late eating. Anticipating that you may have to respond to an alarm at any second as you dine or sitting down for a late-night meal after a series of alarms may cause you to eat at an accelerated rate. Also, the hungrier you are when you sit down for a meal, the more likely you are to eat at a ravenous rate and make poor nutritional choices. The faster you eat, the more likely you are to over-consume because your body has less chance to recognize and inform you that you are full. Without a signal to stop, you're more likely to continue eating until you're about ready to explode. This, of course, applies to everyone in any walk of life.

Our advice is to approach all meals, no matter how hungry you are, like a hazardous materials operation: Slow down and get a good size-up first, develop a prudent strategy and then make your move. Assess the meal and determine what is best, good, bad and ugly. Then fill up on the good stuff and enjoy (in moderation) the less-productive delights. As a performance athlete/firefighter, you need to make these meals work for you. Get the most out of your meals by directing your consumption toward the higher-quality foods and eating at a slower pace.

Tours of duty in the fire service or intense training days should be viewed as days of competition. Therefore, breakfast, lunch and dinner should be viewed as (and therefore designed as) pre-game meals. Pre-game meals should be composed of light and easily digestible, carbohydrate-based foods and quickly absorbable, hydrating beverages. Dining in this manner will productively optimize your state of hydration and top off your muscle and liver glycogen stores. It will also help you to avoid stomach cramps, nausea and the revisiting of your most recent meal. Eating several light meals throughout the day, as opposed to two or three feasts, is most effective in maintaining a healthful blood sugar level and keeping those muscle and liver glycogen stores full. The good food you eat goes right to work, thereby limiting the potential of quality food being converted into fat, as typically occurs with the consumption of super-sized meals.

Simple Truth #6: There are no free lunches.

Pills don't produce training miracles—intelligent training does. It's your hard work and smart consumption, not the inventions of some drug company chemist, that will produce the positive changes you desire. I know what you're thinking: "But professor, the advertisements all seem so genuine and true." You're right, the promises they make do seem fantastic at times. However, when confronted by these sophisticated sales pitches, remember this: If it sounds too good to be true, it probably is. Realize, as the sales pitch continues, that "most of what they tell you is only designed to sell you." Like many a successful politician, those who are pushing magical dietary products are going to tell you anything that they think you want to hear in order to get you to buy their product (or win your vote). Don't become the victim—you're smarter than that. The reality is that by making a few simple adjustments to your current diet, you can obtain all of the nutrients that you need to train intensely, perform at the highest level and enjoy good health.

Chemicals are chemicals: Although some are big and long and others are microscopically small, vitamins, minerals, caffeine, alcohol, steroids and other supplementary ergogenic aids are all just different sorts of ingestible chemicals. When you take chemicals into your body, there will always be an effect. The effects may be good or they may be bad, but long term or short term, there is destined to be a consequence and it may actually be quite adverse. There are no free lunches[6] when it comes to the ingestion of chemical supplements, so *if you don't need'em, don't eat'em*. And guess what—if you consume a well-balanced performance diet focused on nutritious whole foods, chances are you don't need them.

Vitamins are essential for humans to both thrive and survive, hence their original name "vital amines."[9] Plants make them and then we obtain them by either ingesting the plant or some other plant-consuming creature. Of the 13 vitamins that we require, only vitamin D can be substantially produced within the body, so the rest of what we need must be consumed. Vitamins that exist and function in the body's watery fluids are referred to as **water-soluble vitamins**. Those that are stored within our body fat are identified as **fat-soluble vitamins**.

Water-soluble B vitamins play a big role in the breakdown of carbohydrates, proteins and fats to supply energy to working muscles. Given that they are used extensively in energy-releasing (metabolic) reactions, it makes sense that they are abundantly present in the muscles of other animals and fish as well. Consequently, meats, fish and poultry serve as rich sources of B vitamins. For those less inclined to consume the flesh of those featuring "fin, fur and feather,"[14] dairy products, whole grains, and green leafy vegetables are sound alternative choices. Vitamin C is the other key water-soluble vitamin and is important for, among other things, the maintenance of strong bones and cartilage, both of which are critical for high-intensity training and performance. Additionally, vitamin C acts as a powerful antioxidant, assisting the body in its efforts to combat the development of heart disease and cancer, the number one and two killers of Americans and firefighters alike. Citrus fruits (oranges, grapefruit, tangerines, etc.) are a great resource for obtaining vitamin C, as are tomatoes and green leafy vegetables.

Of the fat-soluble vitamins, vitamin A, its precursor beta-carotene and vitamin E all act similarly to vitamin C, functioning as antioxidants to assist the body in neutralizing destructive free radicals. If not defused, circulating free radicals can encourage the development of many serious physiological issues including heart disease and cancer. Consequently, the consumption of foods rich in vitamins A, beta-carotene, C and E is crucial in supporting the body's immune system. Vitamin A also plays an important role in the maintenance of good vision, a critical sense relied upon in firefighting, athletics and other high-performance activities. Vitamin D is principle in the absorption of calcium and the growth and strengthening of bones. Strong bones are necessary to accommodate the stress of intense physical training, dynamic movement, and muscular development. Finally, vitamin K is instrumental in the clotting of blood; something a high-intensity firefighter/athlete knows is key for recovering from intense physical challenges. A variety of green leafy vegetables provide vitamins A, E and K. Fortified milk and other dairy products contain significant amounts of vitamins A and D.

Here are three additional important points relevant to the consumption of vitamins:

- Although the intake of vitamins is essential for the maintenance of good health and productive training, more in the form of supplementation is not necessarily better and too much can cause serious health problems. The excess intake of fat-soluble vitamins in particular can create a hazardous-materials event in your body that results in a variety of serious health issues. This is largely due to the fact that fat-soluble vitamins tend to be stored and can therefore accumulate to toxic levels. You really don't need to get involved with any sort of vitamin or mineral supplementation. Simply maintain the prescribed performance diet and you should be able to obtain all of the vitamins, minerals, water, fiber, fuel, fat and amino acids that you need to support the maintenance of good health, high-intensity training and performance.
- B vitamins are not a source of fuel for the body. They assist with the breakdown of carbohydrate, protein and fat to release energy, but they themselves do not get broken down (metabo-

lized) to release energy. As such, they are used repeatedly and therefore do not need to be replaced as often as those who manufacture and market vitamin supplements would like you to believe.

- Eat foods that contain the necessary vitamins, rather than vitamins packed into a pill. The combined effects of many factors (some known and others not yet undiscovered) seem to provide the healthful and disease prevention benefits associated with vitamins and minerals in foods. So to experience the desired benefits of your nutritional goals, you're probably best off eating the foods that contain the targeted vitamins and minerals rather than taking the pill.

Minerals are also required in amazingly small quantities. The mass sum of all 22 minerals in the body amounts to less than approximately 4 percent of one's total weight.[9] That's about 7 pounds of minerals in the average firefighter who weighs 175 pounds. Still, they're absolutely essential to the maintenance of good health and the execution of high-intensity physical activity. Specifically, calcium and phosphorous help maintain and develop bones. This, of course, is crucial for enabling the performance of intense physical training and dynamic movement. Calcium also plays an important role in the contraction of muscle fibers. Sodium, potassium and chloride contribute to insuring proper body water balance, maintaining sufficient blood volume and providing water for body cooling via sweat. Sodium and potassium also enable muscle contraction and nerve impulse conduction. Zinc, copper, chromium and iron are all intimately involved in the chemical (metabolic) reactions that release energy to contract muscles. Iron plays a very important role in oxygen transport with red blood cells, and magnesium helps to build and repair muscle tissue.

As with vitamins, minerals can be best obtained through the consumption of a well-balanced diet featuring a wide variety of foods. Focus especially on the full spectrum of whole grains, vegetables and fruits, as well as some low-fat dairy products, lean meats and baked or broiled fish. Similar to vitamins, excess mineral intake through supplementation can result in significant health problems. For example, as important as iron is in facilitating the delivery of oxygen as a component of hemoglobin in red blood cells, supplementation of iron beyond that which the body can readily use accumulates and then potentially contributes to the development of heart damage, diabetes, and liver disease as well as possibly encouraging the growth of certain cancers such as colorectal cancer; a particular hazard to firefighters. Furthermore, supplementing with salt tablets in an attempt to replace salt lost via sweat can be hazardous because it may dangerously elevate body salt concentration. Most people void the excess salt they consume in their urine, but those who are sodium intolerant cannot. The storage of excess sodium results in the retention of body water and the potential development of high blood pressure. A point worth noting is that the average American takes in nearly ten times the daily requirement for sodium without ever lifting the salt shaker from the table.[9] Because salts are used extensively in foods as flavor enhancers and preservatives, chances are that the salts you lose in sweating will be replaced with your next meal.

Simple Truth #7: Drink heavily!

The seventh and final simple truth of performance nutrition deems that if you lose a great deal of body water via sweat during a workout or fire, you need to drink a bit more than you lost in order to reestablish your proper level of hydration. Thus, if you sweat like a hog as a consequence of intense physical activity, you would be well advised to drink heavily to replace those precious lost body fluids. To cool your body off, produce energy quickly and transport nutrients and waste products to and from working muscles, you need to maintain an optimal state of hydration. Training will effectively increase your body's capacity to store water and utilize it productively, so all you have to do is provide the essential fluid. Beverages provide most of the fluid in your diet. Fruits and vegetables can also contribute significantly, and a very small quantity of water is additionally obtained as an end product of energy-producing (metabolic) reactions. Acknowledging the importance of peak hydration, and wanting to proactively ensure the maintenance of a well-hydrated state, you need to know a) how to evaluate your state of hydration, b) how much fluid to consume in order to replace measured fluid loss and c) how to most rapidly replace the body fluid you have lost.

Evaluating your state of hydration

The easiest way to determine your current state of hydration, and measure the amount of water you may have lost through physical activity, via sweat, is by weighing yourself. Stepping onto the scale each morning is an excellent way to determine your hydration status at the start of a day. Also, weighing yourself prior to training or work and then again after your training session or fire will enable you to estimate your body water loss and aid you in your efforts to effectively rehydrate.

Everybody sweats at different rates. As an example, we once had two well-conditioned firefighters involved in a training project that were the same age, size and gender, as well as being nearly identical in terms of body composition and aerobic fitness. Interestingly, however, one featured a sweat rate that was a full liter per hour greater than the other: ~2.6/hour vs. ~1.6/hour. Naturally, we called the heavy sweater "Wet-man" and the less prolific secretor "Dry-man." One thing we discovered in a separate study is that when firefighters operate at high intensity in firefighting gear, they sweat at their absolute maximum rate. This may be in excess of three liters per hour![8] Many factors influence your rate of sweating, including genetics, training status, state of hydration, age, gender and body size. We therefore suggest that you measure and determine (by weight) your own personal rate of total body fluid loss rather than guessing and potentially being way off.

Replacing lost body fluid

For each pound of reduced weight that you note in weighing yourself after either a workout or fire, you have lost approximately one pint of body water. For every two pounds, you have lost nearly a quart (or liter). Given that you won't absorb or retain all of the water that you drink to rehydrate, you should always consume a bit more than your weight indicates that you have lost.

The quickest way to replace lost body fluid is by drinking a very cold and watered-down beverage to fill your stomach to about two-thirds of capacity. The colder the fluid, the more rapidly it will move from your stomach to the small intestine, where it can be absorbed. Drinks that feature lower concentrations of any type of sugar, other forms of carbohydrate, protein or fat will also move most rapidly from your stomach down into your small intestine. The natural tendency of the elastic stomach wall to return to its originally smaller size when it is stretched creates a pressure on the stomach fluid, which likely facili-

LAST CALL

Here are a few final recommendations of simple yet powerful dietary actions that you can take to enhance your personal nutrition and therefore health, appearance and performance.

1. **Raisin Bran for Breakfast:** Possibly the simplest way for firefighters to most profoundly influence their health and performance through diet would be to drop the fried eggs, bacon and donuts at breakfast in favor of a bowl of raisin bran or other similarly nutritious brand of cereal. Given the low-fat nature and rich carbohydrate, vitamin, mineral and fiber content of this choice meal, you'll be fueling up and cleaning out your body wisely rather than clogging it up and filling it with slow-burning fuel.

2. **Fruit for Snacks:** You may never be quite as popular as the coworker who brings in the donuts, pastries, cake or ice cream, but you'll be contributing in a positive way to all of your coworkers lives when you bring in a nice selection of fresh fruit instead of the lard-ladened alternatives. If you clean it up and put it in a bowl at the center of the table, it'll be gone in no time flat. And again, rather than clogging up and slowing them down, you'll be fueling them up and cleaning them out. The fuel, vitamin, mineral, water and fiber content in fruits are enormous.

3. **Add a Colorful Salad:** Along the same lines as fruit, the addition of a salad to your lunch or dinner is an absolute home run. The quantity of healthful nutrients (vitamins, minerals, fuel, water and fiber) in a colorful salad is huge. If you serve up a salad prior to the main course, everyone wins: filling up on the good stuff makes you less inclined to eat too much of any subsequent suboptimal selections. As a general rule, the more diverse the selection of colors in your salad, the more varied the vitamin and mineral content. One word of warning, though: Always apply your own salad dressing so that you can limit the amount applied. A tasteful sprinkling of low-fat dressing is definitely the way to go. Adding a lot of fatty dressing to your salad is essentially the same as serving it deep-fried. What kind of sense does that make? It's like fumbling in the end zone, or intercepting a pass and running the wrong way. It's something very good gone terribly wrong!

4. **Go Fish:** Given the extremely high rates of heart disease among Americans and firefighters in particular, it makes good sense to consume baked or broiled deep-sea fish about twice a week. This will provide you with a healthful supply of cardio-protective omega-3 fatty acids. Salmon, sardines and shell fish are a few select choices. But remember, in frying the fish you destroy the dish (from a health perspective).

tates its forward movement down into the intestine. Casually walking around as you rehydrate may be of benefit as this mechanical movement seems to encourage the transfer of fluid from the stomach to small intestine. If it's necessary to continue with your rehydration efforts, drink an additional six to eight ounces every 10 to 15 minutes.

To optimize your state of hydration, concentrate on maintaining a carbohydrate-rich diet featuring plenty of fruits and vegetables. Additionally, you should drink plenty of water and juices and minimize your intake of caffeinated and alcoholic beverages.

Flexibility Training

You just smoked another killer circuit with the weights. You're shot, but you feel good. You won every battle, pushing through the pain and fatigue to get it done. Your arms are so exhausted that you subconsciously elect to lean on the door rather than push it open as you exit the gym. You grin as you think to yourself, "Another great session in the bank." Walking to the showers, you stop for a drink from the fountain; the cool water feels good in your dry mouth. You're preoccupied in thought, reviewing your last few workouts. It's always an enjoyable activity, kind of like counting money in the bank. You're thinking, "One hundred and one floors on the Stairmaster yesterday, a full weight-training circuit the day before, Monday was a nice 5K run through the park....Hey, what's missing here?"

Flexibility training (stretching) is clearly the ugly stepchild of the fitness family—uniquely important but tragically neglected. Almost every athlete has a sense of its value and importance, yet too often it just doesn't seem to get done. Why? Well, there are probably a thousand plausible excuses, but the real reason in most cases is that it's just a lot easier *not* to do it. Unfortunately, if you're involved in rigorous physical training and you don't routinely stretch, you are unquestionably limiting your athletic potential and setting yourself up for serious injury. For high-intensity firefighter/athletes in particular, a comprehensive routine of consistent stretching is essential.

Whether you're positively developing muscle tissue through training or de-conditioning (atrophying) muscle as a consequence of inactivity, muscle tissue responds similarly—it tends to shorten. Shortened muscles results in reduced range of motion and impaired movement. If you attempt to stretch that shortened muscle beyond the point where it can now comfortably and safely go, it's going to tear. Whether the tear is microscopic or pronounced, the consequence is in essence the same: injury.

Inflexibility leads to inevitable injury. With high-performance firefighter/athletes in particular, it is only a question of "when," not "if," the muscle strain (or worse) will occur. When your range of motion becomes compromised, the next door you force, the next ceiling you pull, the next athletic cut you take or the next strenuous lift you make will likely result in significant soft tissue (muscle, tendon or ligament) injury.

The good news is that an ounce of prevention is worth a ton of rehab. Even a small commitment on your part to routinely stretch can markedly reduce your potential for soft tissue injury and enhance your athletic or fire field performance. Just five to ten minutes of painless effort per day is all it takes. Naturally, you can take this type of training as far as you'd like; however, to reap the most important gains you merely need to stretch for a brief period each day. You don't have to stretch to the point of being able to tie yourself into knots. All you need to do is stretch properly, consistently and comprehensively.

Stretching techniques and programs, just like every other form of physical training, are offered in many different shapes and colors. Pilates and yoga, for instance, are two excellent and popular flexibility-enhancing activities. The trick here, though, is to find a method that is safe, effective and, most of all, useful for you. Our recommendation is to try a form of flexibility training called static stretching. Static stretching has been used successfully by athletes since the days of the dinosaurs, just prior to my birth. It's not exactly the new kid on the flexibility training block, but it's certainly the most popular. It's the preferred method of flexibility training among sports professionals and trainers worldwide for two good reasons: it's very safe to use and proven to be effective. It works well with any level of physical ability and requires no special equipment so you can begin as soon as you'd like. The program we have developed engages all of the body's major muscle groups in one logical and easy-to-use set of stretching movements. Routine completion of this comprehensive fire-oriented stretching routine will significantly improve your overall flexibility, dynamic movement, physical performance and job safety.

Training Benefits

In addition to the many benefits mentioned, progressive and consistent flexibility training through static stretching can result in:

- Improved circulation
- Improved posture and balance of opposing muscle
- Decreased risk of lower back pain and sciatica
- Reduced stress

For the firefighter, improved coordination and balance that results from safe and effective flexibility programming can be life saving as well as performance enhancing. Its need is apparent in the execution of critical job tasks such as climbing ladders, entering windows, and crawling through confined spaces. If you're having trouble getting through a window off a fire escape because your hamstrings are too tight, you're making a hazardous job a heck of a lot more dangerous. Imagine what is likely to happen to that hamstring when you force your way out in a hurry with fire right at your back—you're a "lock" for a hamstring tear. Why add unnecessary consequence to the perilous efforts you make? The same fundamental truth applies in other athletic and training settings that involve dynamic movement; a lack of flexibility hampers performance and encourages injury, while good flexibility improves health, safety and performance.

Improved flexibility can be achieved by anyone, but like anything else that eventually results in success, it requires conscientious effort and consistent practice. Although neglected by a great many athletes, flexibility training (stretching) is a clear and essential component of fitness training that needs to be emphasized in any legitimate fitness or athletic training program. High-performance firefighter/athletes must therefore realize that flexibility training is a critical element of their comprehensive training program and *just do it*!

Firefighter I Flexibility Program

The Firefighter I Flexibility Program, organized in a progressive and easy-to-use manner, is composed of 16 basic exercises running in series from the lower legs and progressing upward through the body to the neck. Firefighter/athletes should complete the Firefighter I Flexibility Training Program prior to the beginning of their tour of duty, and before any athletic event or training session. Casually and comfortably completing the full flexibility set at the conclusion of a training session is also an excellent way to cool down after a rigorous workout; additional stretching can be done at any time. Use these stretches throughout the day to keep yourself ready at all times. For those of you sitting behind a desk, periodic stretching can actually be a re-energizing event. Break free of your bondage to the computer screen and for just a few moments engage in some good light stretching. It'll wake you up and help to prevent annoying joint stiffness and muscle soreness.

The step-by-step instructions we've provided on the following pages will enable you to learn the program quickly. Perform all of the stretches we've listed to ensure that you involve your entire musculoskeletal system. In doing so, you'll achieve increased functional flexibility, suppleness, strength and control in movement, as well as improved balance, mobility and coordination.

All the stretches can be easily performed in the firehouse with the use of the rig or at home with the use of a chair or any other immovable object. To get the most out of your stretch, you need to relax. Sometimes this is a bit of a challenge for high-intensity humans, but it's absolutely facilitative and therefore very important. Once you've relaxed and set yourself into the *initial position*, you can begin. Follow the easy-to-use static stretching protocol (see box) that we've developed for you. Work your way through the Firefighter I program at your own pace, paying particular attention to body positions and movements as you learn the new stretches. Then simply enjoy the benefits of your enhanced flexibility.

Additional Points & Recommendations:

- **Stretch only to the point where you feel mild tension.** In order to get the most out of your stretches, move into the stretch in a steady and relaxed manner. If you move too quickly, push or bounce into the stretch, a defensive reflex will actually cause the stretching muscles to contract. This is counter-productive and potentially injurious. Interestingly, the muscle, when dramatically stretched, reflexively contracts in an effort to try and protect itself from being torn apart.

- **Avoid stretching to the point where numbness or a tingling sensation is felt.** If you begin to feel numbness or tingling, you're probably affecting the nerve or nerves adjacent to the muscle being stretched. Back off a little and maintain a position in the stretch that doesn't cause the undesirable sensation.
- **Focus and try to relax the muscles involved in the stretch.** Relaxing the involved muscles throughout the passive movement of the stretch will aid in alleviating any unnecessary tension within the muscles. Using the principles of opposites, the muscle being stretched needs to remain relaxed. This will result in increased flexibility in the muscles and connective tissues, and yield quicker adaptation to the stretching program.
- **Do NOT hold your breath! Breathe in a slow, comfortable and controlled manner.** It's common to hold your breath when you're stressed or swimming under water. However, it's *not* a good practice when performing your stretching routine. Breathe in a slow and controlled manner to promote relaxation and facilitate the stretching movement. Always exhale for the first few seconds as you are performing the movement. Then breathe in a slow, comfortable and controlled manner as you hold the stretch. Inhale as you return to the initial position.
- **Hold all stretches for at least 15 seconds.** The recommended time frame of 15 to 20 seconds is derived from research on the effect of static stretch on athletic performance. This is enough time to disengage the stretch reflex that actually contracts muscles in an attempt to protect against overstretching.

STATIC STRETCHING PROTOCOL

1. Place yourself into the initial position for the stretch.
2. Exhale and move slowly, smoothly and gently into the stretch.
3. Continue into the stretch, moving to the point where you feel mild tension (not pain), and then stop.
4. Maintain the "static stretch" position for 15 to 20 seconds, breathing freely, easily and slowly.
5. If you feel comfortable at this point, you may move slightly deeper into the stretch.
6. Hold the final "static position" for another 15 to 20 seconds and then slowly return to the initial position.

1. Motor Pump Operator (MPO) Stretches

Target: Gastrocnemius, soleus, Achilles tendon

These stretches can also be done with a chair or wall.

Straight-leg MPO Stretch

Position: Place your hands on the bumper of the rig (or wall) and stand with your feet about shoulder-width apart, one foot forward and the other foot back; both feet face forward. Bend your front knee and move your hips forward, keeping your back leg straight and your back heel flat on the ground.

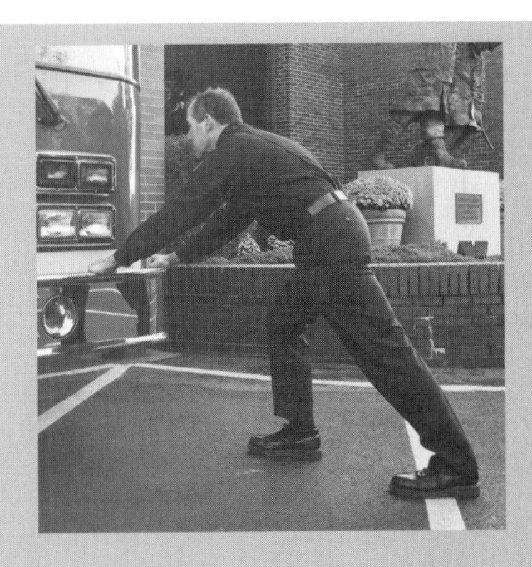

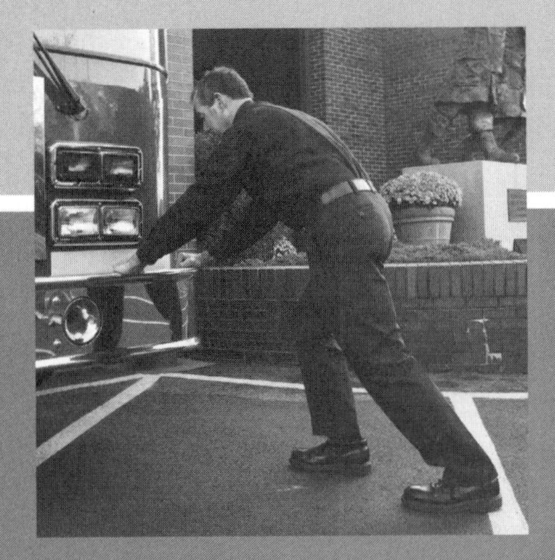

Bent-leg MPO Stretch

Position: Place your hands on the bumper of the rig (or wall) and stand with your feet about shoulder-width apart, one foot forward and the other foot back; both feet face forward. Bend both knees slightly, moving your hips forward while keeping your back heel flat on the ground.

2. Roofman's Stretch

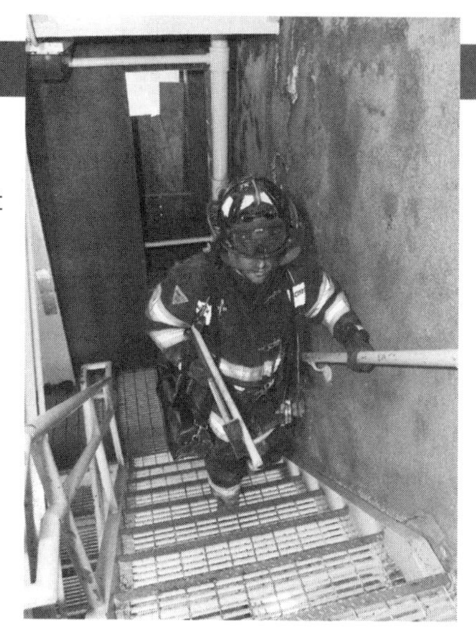

Target: Quadriceps

Position: Place one hand on the rig (or wall) and hold the ankle furthest from the rig with the same-side hand. Pull your heel toward your gluteal muscles.

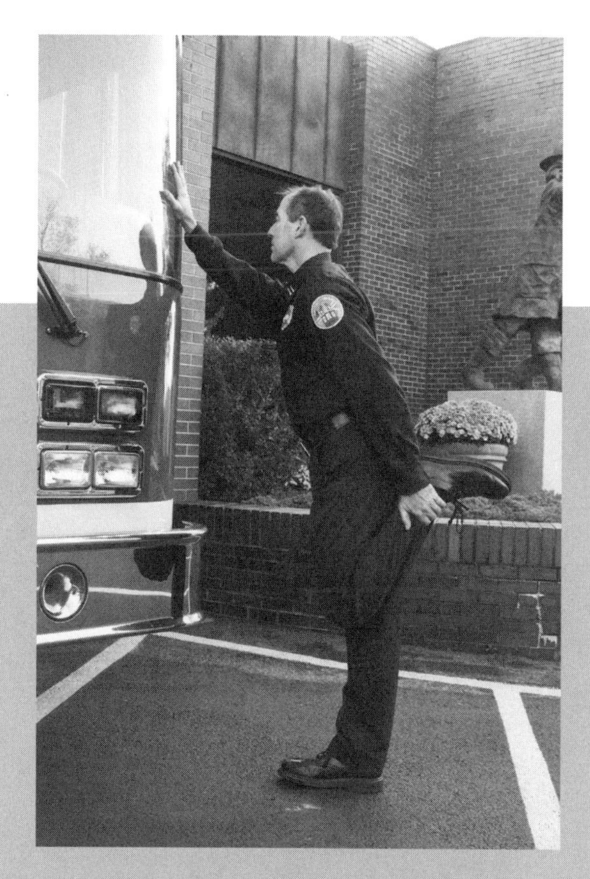

3. Chauffeur's Stretches

Target: Hamstrings

Straight-leg Chauffeur's Stretch

Position: Raise one leg onto the bumper of the rig (or chair), keeping the raised leg straight. Bend forward at the hip, moving your chest toward your raised leg without bending your knee.

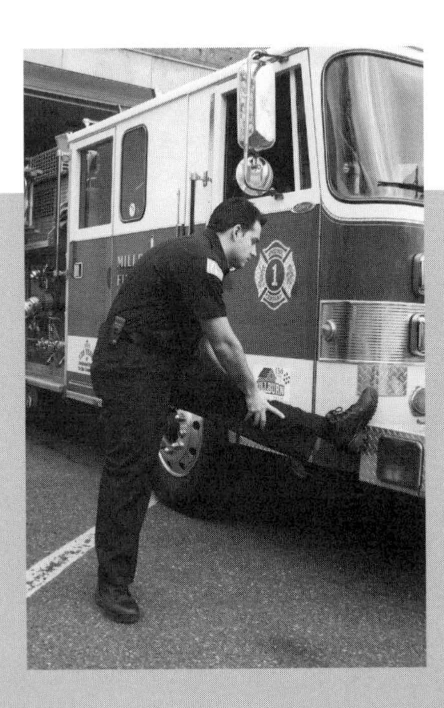

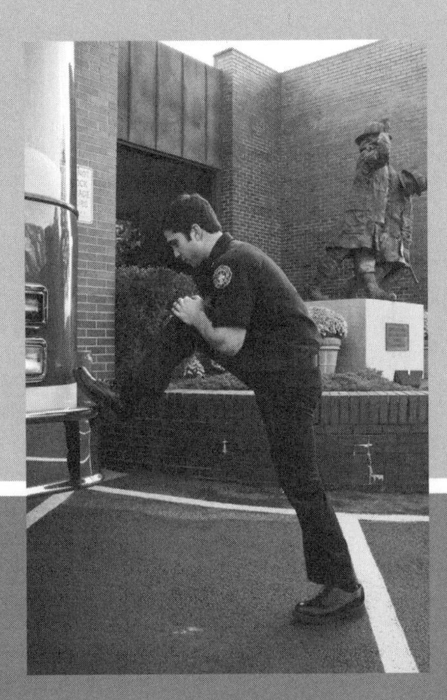

Bent-leg Chauffeur's Stretch

Target: hip flexors, groin, gluteals

Position: Place one foot on the bumper of the rig (or chair) with your knee bent. Your back leg should be slightly bent and your front leg should be turned slightly outward. Lean forward, moving your hips toward the rig (or chair).

4. Outside Vent Man's Reach & Twist

Target: Latissimus dorsi, trunk flexors

Reach

Position: Stand with your feet about shoulder-width apart and knees slightly bent. Holding a hook (or rope) with your hands slightly more than shoulder-width apart, extend your arms overhead. Lean to one side and then the other.

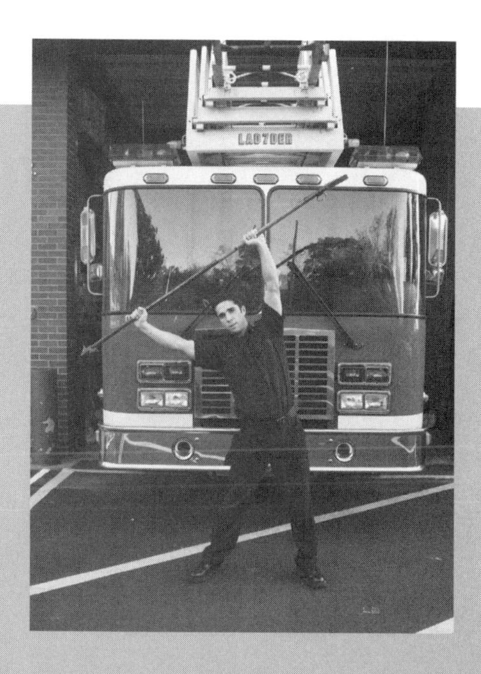

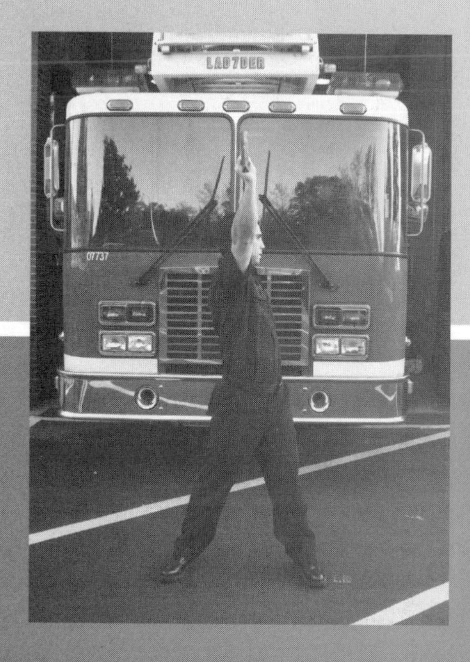

Twist

Position: Stand with your feet about shoulder-width apart and knees slightly bent. Holding a hook (or rope) with your hands slightly more than shoulder-width apart, extend your arms overhead. Twist in one direction and then the other.

5. Controlman's Stretch

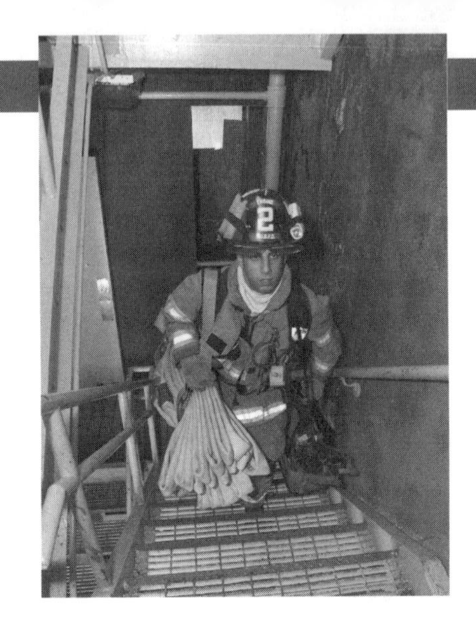

Target: Hamstrings, lower back

Position: Stand with your feet about shoulder-width apart and your hands resting on the bumper of the rig (or chair). Bend at the hips, keeping your back flat and knees straight.

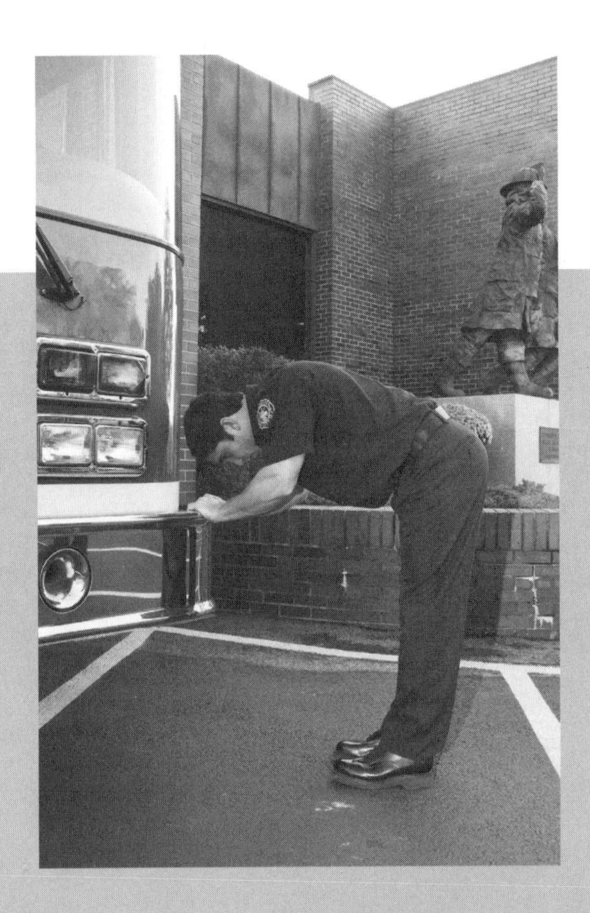

6. Forcible Entry Team Stretches

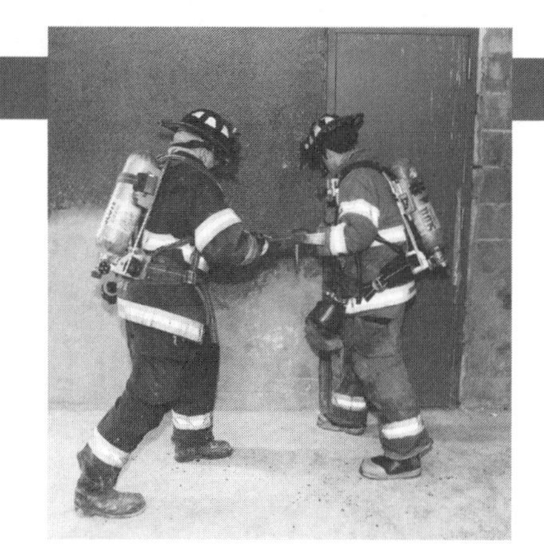

Target: Pectorals

Pec Stretch

Position: Standing sideways to the rig (or wall), bend your arm into an "L" shape and place it on the rig. Place one foot in front of the other. Slowly turn your body away from the rig (or wall).

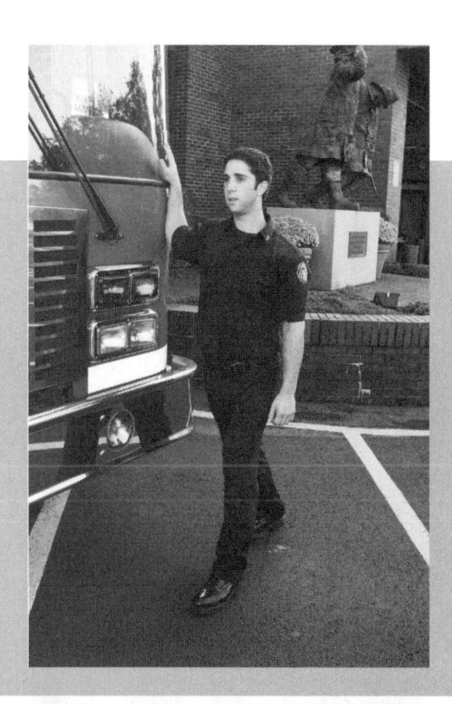

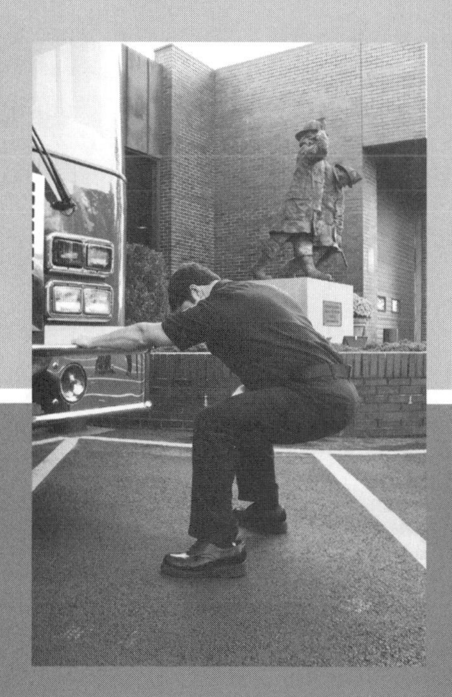

Lat Stretch

Target: Latissimus dorsi

Position: Hold the rig bumper (or some other immovable object) with one hand. Your feet should be about shoulder-width apart and your knees should be bent into a squatting position. Lean back slightly.

7. Housewatchman's Stretch

Target: Anterior and posterior deltoids

Front

Position: Stand with your feet about shoulder-width apart. Clasp your hands together behind your back with your elbows slightly bent. Extend and then lift your arms.

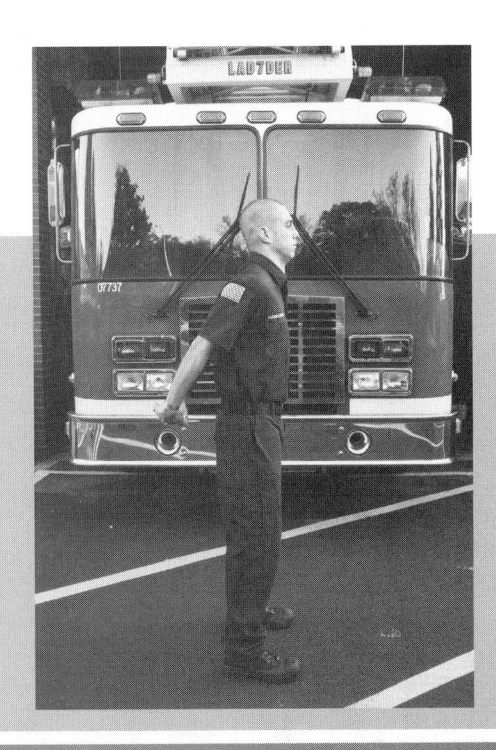

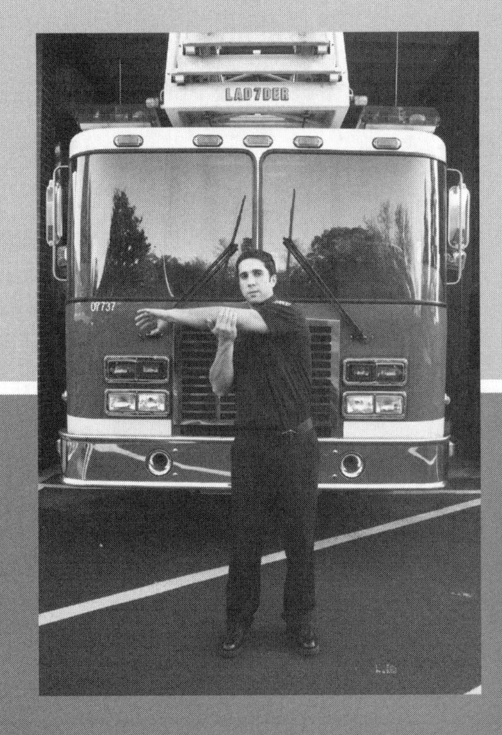

Back

Position: Stand with your feet about shoulder-width apart and hold your left arm across your chest. Place your right hand on your left triceps and press the arm inward. Pull your arm inward.

8. Nozzleman's Stretch

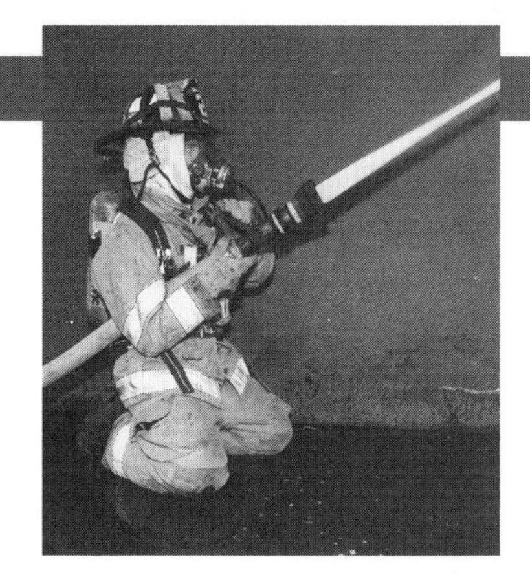

Target: Biceps

Position: Extend your arm to your side at shoulder height and grasp the rig (or wall). Turn your body away from the rig (or wall).

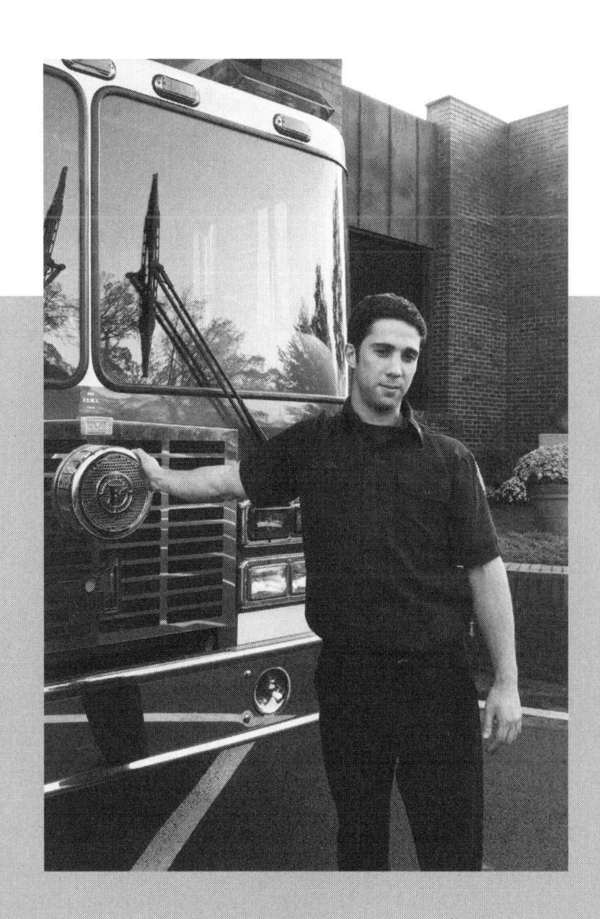

9. Ironman's Stretch

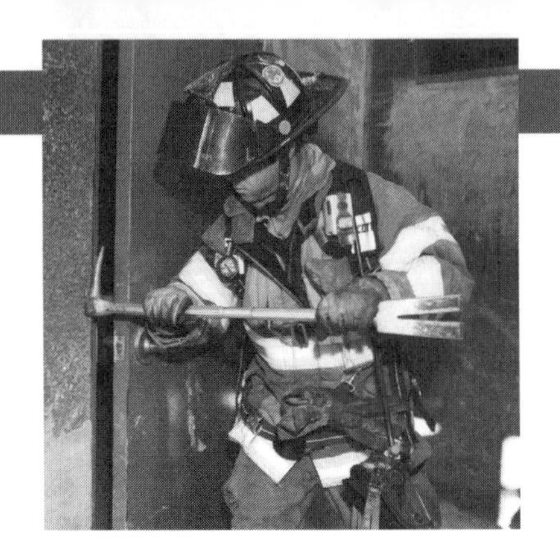

Target: Triceps

Position: Stand with your feet about shoulder-width apart. Bend one arm behind your head, holding your elbow with the other hand. Gently push the elbow back and down.

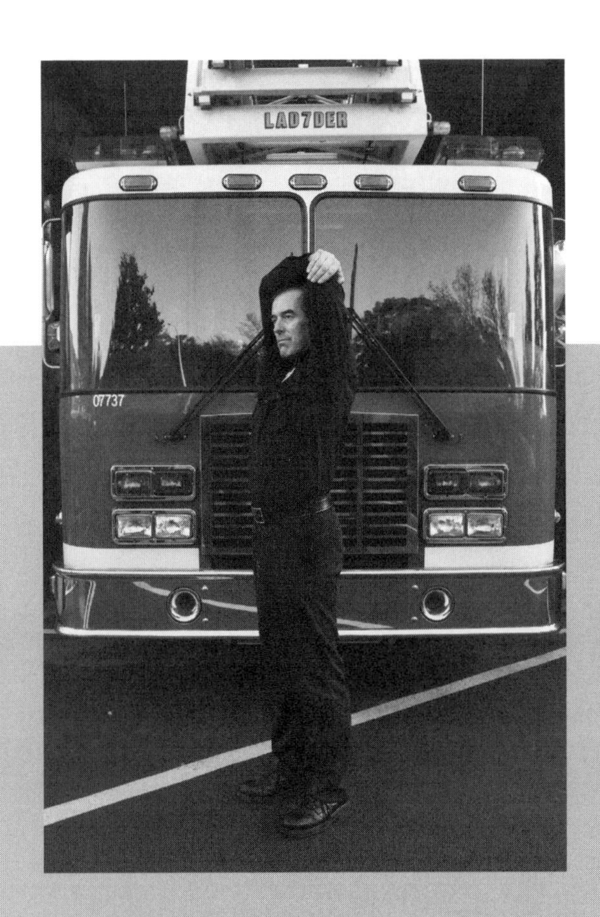

10. Tillerman's Stretch

Target: Sternocleidomastoid, trapezius

Side

Position: Stand with your feet about shoulder-width apart and grasp the left side of your head with your right hand. Pull your head gently toward your right shoulder.

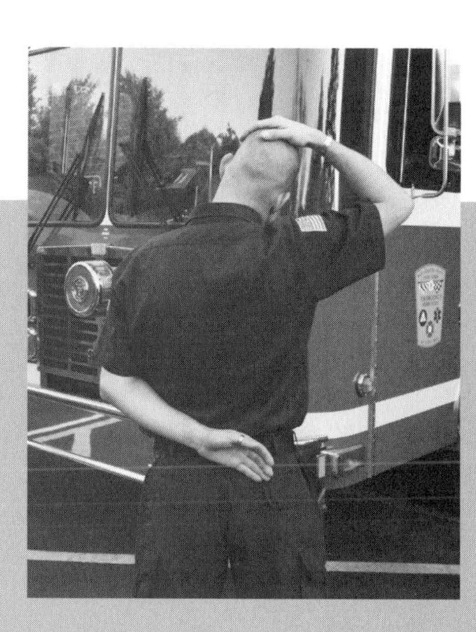

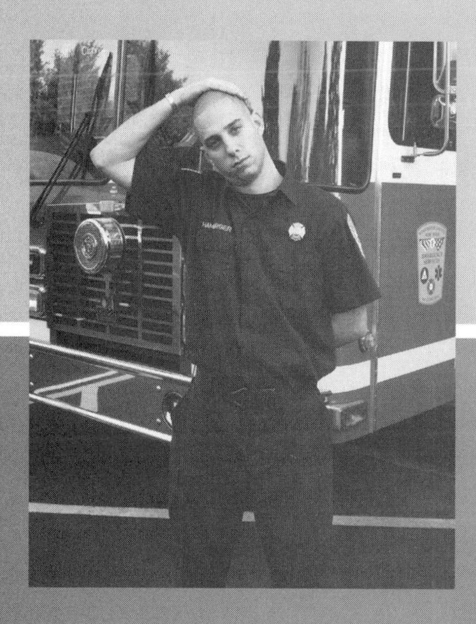

Diagonal

Position: Stand with your feet about shoulder-width apart and grab behind your left ear with your right hand. Pull your head gently toward your right armpit.

Aerobic Training

Simply stated, aerobic fitness is the foundation of firefighter performance. The more oxygen firefighters can take in, transport, deliver and utilize to produce energy, the harder they can work, the more work they can do and the quicker they can recover from strenuous tasks. Firefighters who are aerobically fit are able to ascend stairs more rapidly and recover more swiftly to force entry and rescue victims or extinguish fire. To complete such critical tasks in the shortest time possible, firefighter/athletes must achieve and maintain a high level of aerobic fitness.

Every fire serves to remind firefighters just how important aerobic fitness is to their performance and survival—the more frequent or intense the reminder, the more indelible the mark. This makes it perhaps a little easier for firefighters in busy fire companies to maintain a high level of motivation to train. However, every firefighter needs to be prepared at all times because when the bell rings, the potential always exists for maximal demands in a life-threatening situation.

The extraordinary acts of firefighters working at the New York City World Trade Center Operation on September 11, 2001, demonstrated the incredibly beneficial effects of aerobic conditioning on firefighter work performance. To affect the search-and-rescue efforts necessary to successfully remove thousands of victims from within the twin towers, firefighters had to forcefully ascend countless flights of stairs in full gear, carrying their tools and equipment. They had to search, locate, attend to and then either assist out or carry down scores of injured civilians. Acknowledging the dangers but understanding fully the urgency of their work, fiercely tough firefighters continued to climb in an effort to save more lives. Thousands of people were rescued and successfully evacuated as a result of the incredible efforts of these fit, knowledgeable and courageous individuals. Their selfless commitment and heroic efforts were perhaps best represented through the words of Captain Patrick Brown of Ladder 3 in his communication from the North Tower. After reporting on the grim status of the situation on floor 35, he stated with great focus and determination, in the manner of a consummate professional, that he and his fellow firefighters were "still heading up." Every firefighter's capacity was tested as they accomplished the incomprehensible feat of saving thousands of innocent people's lives.

Training Benefits

Consistent aerobic training can produce a wide variety of health and performance benefits. It develops all of the body components and processes involved with the intake, transport, delivery and use of oxygen. Additionally, it enhances your body's cooling system, as well as your abilities to store important carbohydrate fuel, burn fat and regulate blood sugar. In just a few weeks you're going to look better, feel better, perform better and possibly even sleep better. And as if that weren't enough, you'll even bolster your body's defense to prevent such diseases as cancer, diabetes, heart disease, hypertension and obesity. It's almost too good to be true, but the fact is that you can obtain all of these phenomenal health and performance benefits for as little as the cost of a decent pair of running sneakers. Once you've got the sneakers, all you have to do is develop your plan of action and get out the door. Don't you wish all things in life were so simple?

For those of you who'd like a more comprehensive description of the many possible benefits of consistent and progressive aerobic training, a detailed listing is provided below.

- Increases the amount of air you breathe in and out of your lungs with each breath and the maximum amount of air you breathe during high-intensity activity.
- Enhances your ability to move oxygen from your lungs into your blood and remove carbon dioxide.
- Increases the amount of blood as well as the number of vessels in your body in order to transport oxygen and nutrients to working muscle and carry away carbon dioxide.
- Increases the number of oxygen-carrying red blood cells in your blood and the amount of a special compound inside your muscle that shuttles oxygen during energy release.
- Increases your heart's ability to pump out more blood with each beat and, most importantly, during maximum-intensity exercise.
- Increases the size of aerobic (type I) muscle fibers.
- Increases the size and number of energy-producing mitochondria within the muscle cell as well as the number of enzymes in the muscle cell responsible for producing aerobic energy.
- Increases your ability to store glycogen (carbohydrate) as fuel in the muscle cell.
- Increases the number of high-energy-storing molecules within the muscle fiber.
- Increases your ability to produce aerobic energy without the generation of lactic acid during high-intensity exercise and enhances your ability to tolerate fatigue-causing lactic acid.
- Increases your total body water and the number and capacity of your sweat glands.
- Enhances the distribution of sweat, improves the efficiency of cooling, and improves your sweat reaction (you'll sweat earlier in response to exercise).
- Decreases the total amount of heart disease–causing cholesterol in your blood by decreasing the number of LDL (bad cholesterol) proteins, which deposit heart disease–causing cholesterol on the walls of your arteries; and by increasing the number of HDL (good cholesterol) proteins, which pick up and dispose of unwanted cholesterol.
- Decreases the amount of unhealthy fats in the blood as well as unwanted total body fat.
- Decreases blood pressure during exercise and rest.
- Improves your ability to move sugar from your blood to inside your muscle.
- Reduces the potential to develop certain forms of cancer.

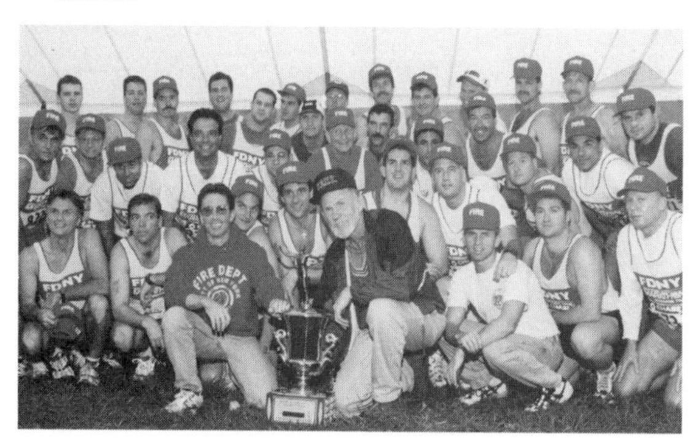

Aerobic Program

You can attain the level of aerobic fitness necessary to perform at the height of your physical work capacity by applying our prescribed aerobic training methods and committing to the process of consistent, progressive and intelligent training. Read, learn and employ the following aerobic training principles to formulate your personal training strategy, achieve your training goals and enjoy the success of your labors.

Developing Your Personalized Training Program

1. Select your personal goal.

In order to develop your personal aerobic training program, you must decide exactly what it is that you ultimately want to achieve. It may be a relatively simply goal like getting out for a light 20-minute jog three days a week or it may be to run a marathon in under three hours. Once you've identified your primary goal, you can work to develop a gradual and progressive training program that'll get you there. Try to be realistic in your goal selection. If your primary goal involves major improvements, it's a good idea to create a progressive series of short-term goals to lead you there.

2. Engage in training specificity.

The second thing you need to do is select the best type of exercise to get you from where you are to where you want to go. If your goal is to simply train aerobically for 20 minutes three times a week in order to reduce body fat and obtain general physical and physiological benefits, then the best form of aerobic exercise for you is the form you most enjoy (or dislike least). Logically, people are much more likely to exercise more frequently and for longer duration if they use a type of exercise that they actually enjoy.

If you aspire to run a marathon, selecting an exercise type is quite simple and straightforward. If you're looking to improve your CPAT time or overall capacity to fight fires, however, the field of effective aerobic exercises becomes much more diverse. Stairclimbing, running, rowing and cycling would all be excellent aerobic training choices, contributing positively in slightly different ways. In the case of training to be Firefighter Fit, the use of more than one type of exercise may actually be most productive. Some firefighter/athletes have been very successful using all four. In simple terms, the objective here is to select and use the right exercises to develop the capacity of the right muscles the right way.

3. Train consistently.

Consistent training is the absolute key to aerobic conditioning success. In order to progress and improve, more than anything else you must first work to develop a consistent training routine. Once this has been achieved, you're well on your way; you can develop a solid training base and then slowly and progressively increase the duration (time or distance) and intensity of your workouts. However, the first priority is to find the best way for you to fit aerobic training into your life. Our recommendations in this regard are to select a most realistic time of day to train and to keep your initial training sessions short and easy.

Depending upon your life schedule and training goals, it may be best for you to start out with just three training sessions a week. This is an excellent way for many people to begin, especially those who lead busy lives. If this describes you, just be certain to hit these three important workouts each week. This will help you to establish a solid training routine and develop a strong training foundation. Then, if or when you decide to, you can always build from there.

The most productive way to obtain the full spectrum of desirable benefits and perform at your full potential as a result of aerobic training is to build to the point where you're training essentially every day. The length and intensity of workouts should vary to maintain a productive training balance, but the ultimate goal with aerobic training should be to try and get out and do it everyday. Your life schedule may not permit you to make this type of commitment and, in fact, your training goals may be focused more in another direction; however, to perform on the level of a high-intensity firefighter, you'll ultimately need to build to the point of training nearly every day, and frequently at higher intensities and for longer durations.

Reversibility: The down side to missing a few days (for whatever reason) of training is that once you go beyond 72 hours, the body moves from a beneficial mode of rehabilitation, reconstruction and enhancement to the clearly less desirable mode of deconstruction and deconditioning. That's right—after just three days of sedentary existence (living like a lump instead of an athlete), you regrettably start to de-condition. This is the real-life application of the fateful training expression "if you don't use it, you lose it." Therefore, try your best to stay on track. Keep in mind that even a short, light workout is often better than no training at all. With beginners in particular, it's very important to minimize the number of goose eggs (0 miles) on the training chart.[3]

4. Build Gradual, Intelligent Progressions.

Consistent aerobic training will provide your cells, muscles, tissues, organs and systems with an overload stimulus that can produce very constructive gains. The term "cardiovascular overload" may sound a little scary, but it's just a phrase used to describe a training intensity that is somewhat greater than that which your body is currently used to. If properly applied, it can rapidly provide outstanding health and performance gains. The key is to overload the cardiovascular system in the same intelligent, well-balanced, gradual and progressive manner as you would other muscles, tissues and systems to generate improvement. In developing your personalized training progression with a particular mode of exercise, you'll need to consider the manipulation of three important conditioning variables: training frequency, duration and intensity.

Training Frequency: The "cookbook" prescription for obtaining aerobic training effect is to exercise three times per week for 20 minutes or more at moderate intensity. If you abide by that training doctrine, you're bound to realize genuine training improvements within a short period of time, especially if you're starting from a relatively low fitness level. This is a well-established fact. However, it has been our experience that many people who train with the use of a three-day-a-week routine often fail because the concept of skipping days tends to lead toward missing weeks and

BASELINE 20-MINUTE EXERCISE SESSION

This workout can be shortened on days when your training time is very limited, or lengthened as your fitness improves. Just remember to always include both a warm-up and cool-down composed of light stretching and 3–5 minutes of comfortably paced walking. The main body of the workout should involve a combination of jogging and walking. As you progress, your jogging intervals will gradually increase. Ultimately, you'll build to the point of being able to run for the entire 10 minutes.

- **Warm up:** Start out by walking for about 5 minutes at a comfortable pace to effectively warm up your body for the slightly more intense jog ahead.
- **Exercise:** Begin your jog, moving at a slow and easy pace. Continue running for as long as you feel comfortable. As soon as you begin to feel fatigued, out of breath or any cramping, slow your pace down to a walk. Continue walking at a casual pace until you feel comfortable and completely recovered. Then resume jogging and continue as before. Alternate between jogging and walking for approximately 10 minutes.
- **Cool down:** Finish up by walking at a comfortable pace for the final 5 minutes of the session.

then months. We recommend that you try to build toward the ultimate goal of participating in your selected form of aerobic training (to some extent) every day. The key to success lies in breaking the psychological barrier between non-training and training through the development of a brief, easy and consistent (daily, rather than periodic) training routine. Make some workout days shorter than others if necessary in order to get something in every day. Once you've developed this kind of frequency in training, you're a shoe-in for success and you can build to the sky.

If this is your first attempt at aerobic training, we urge you to be patient. Start out with slow and easy workouts. Beginning with light sessions of combined walking and jogging is generally a very good idea. (See the sample 20-minute workout.) Training sessions need to be as enjoyable as possible and short enough to fit easily into your busy day. Once you have gotten off the ground, you should try to build from three workout days to five, six or seven days a week. This consistency in training will produce undeniably positive results, even in the first few weeks.

Training Duration: Frequent and consistent training will in short order produce a rock-solid foundation of conditioning from which you can safely and effectively build. Once the training base has been established, you can begin to slightly increase either the time or distance of your training efforts. Play it smart; make your increases relatively small and only apply them to a couple of workouts each week. Listen to your body and respond to its aches, pains and positive adaptations. As your body improves in response to the gradual increases, you can slowly and progressively continue to build. Just be careful not to overdo it. Many runners suffer overuse injuries such as shin splints and tendonitis at this stage of their training because they increase the duration of their workouts and weekly mileage too dramatically. They do too much too soon and, because the body cannot develop and repair itself fast enough to keep pace with the imposed stress of training, damage mounts and injury results. Early successes often inspire overzealous behavior, leading to regrettably avoidable injuries. Don't become a victim of your own successes. Grant your body the time it needs to respond in a positive way to the physical and physiological training stimulus. If provided with the proper nutrients and given sufficient time to work, the body will do amazing things. Just keep your cool, listen to your body and continue to train smart.

With all aerobic activities, and in particular running, it's common for people to have trouble increasing the duration, distance or time of their workouts. In general, this is because the intensity at which they exercise is much too high; they either run, cycle or swim at too vigorous a pace. You are not going to have this problem because we're going to tip you off to the runner's paradox. It goes something like this: "If you want to run fast, you have to learn to run long

Interestingly, running too fast too soon is why so many people blow their race in the initial mile of the 26.22-mile NYC Marathon. The first mile of the race involves a steady climb up the southern end of the Varrazano Narrows Bridge. Caught up in the overwhelming excitement of the electrifying start in this enormously popular race, many runners either go out too fast or zigzag all over the place trying to get around other slower runners. These actions result in the inefficient combustion of carbohydrate fuel and premature depletion of their essential carbohydrate stores. This will leave them high and dry in Harlem, causing them to "hit the wall" several miles from the finish line at Central Park's Tavern on the Green.

Each year, I'd line up in the second row of the race along with a couple of hundred other FDNY and NYPD runners. At the sound of the cannon, I'd go out pretty quickly for about 50 to 100 meters and then immediately drift over toward the curb. Off to the side and out from the pathway of stampeding runners, I'd adjust my pace to establish a comfortable and efficient rhythm. In the meantime, every runner and his mother would be soaring by, some wearing bunny ears and others connected together in a caterpillar-like chain. The spectacle was hilarious, but not so for the more serious runners who got tragically pulled along with the tide. For these folks it was going to be a long hard day. They would never be able to replace the carbohydrate that they unintentionally and inefficiently spent. By the time I reached the two-mile mark on the far side of the bridge, there would typically be well over a thousand runners ahead of me who had gone out too fast. On good days, I would spend the next two and a half hours reeling them in. I'm no different than anyone else, though; I learned this same lesson the hard way in the Montreal Marathon, where I wound up walking most of the last eight miles. It's the kind of lesson that you don't want to learn twice. To achieve your personal peak performance, you'll need to run smart from the start and tough to the end.

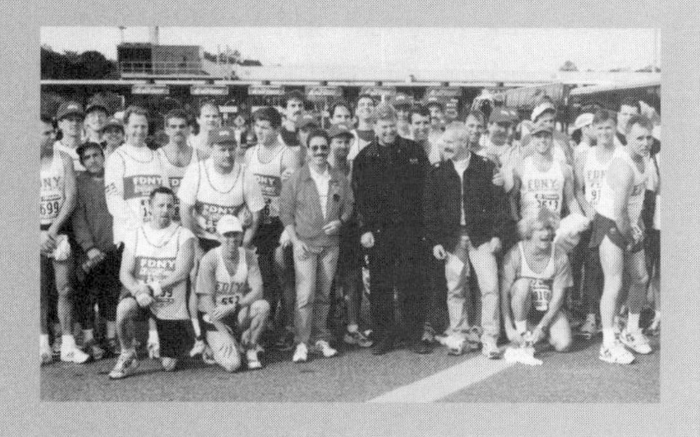

MONITORING YOUR HEART RATE

One very easy way to monitor and regulate your aerobic training intensity and pace is to measure your heart rate. Heart rate measurements can be obtained manually (where you feel your pulse) or they may be measured with the use of a portable monitoring ensemble, such as a chest strap and wrist watch. You can measure your heart rate by taking your pulse at two key locations on your body.

Radial Pulse: Turn the palm of one hand up toward the ceiling. Place the fingertips of the index and middle fingers of the other hand on the wrist, just below the thumb, of the first hand. Feel for the pulse. The radial location provides an accurate measurement of heart rate in most cases.

Carotid Pulse: Place the index and middle fingers of one hand on your neck between the muscles of your neck and throat. Gently feel for the pulse. Be careful not to press too hard on the carotid artery. If you've been exercising vigorously, a strong pulse should be felt.

When taking your pulse at either of these locations, you'll need access to a watch or clock that measures seconds with a sweeping hand or digital display. When you begin to feel the beats with your fingers, start counting from 0, making sure to observe the seconds. A common method is to count your pulse for 10 seconds. Take the number of beats and multiply by 6 to determine your pulse count for one minute. Note that the longer you count the beats, the more accurate the measurement.

The easiest way to measure your heart rate during an exercise session is to simply stop exercising for a moment and then take the measure as described above. This is a very good way to monitor the intensity at which you are training, to see if you are exercising too hard, too easy or at just the right pace. Running at any pace results in the productive expenditure of energy, but to obtain positive cardiovascular training effects through your aerobic conditioning, you should ideally run at a pace that produces a heart rate response of between 70 to 90 percent of your predicted maximum heart rate. Running at a pace that produces a heart rate response of between 70 to 85 percent is particularly effective because it will enable you to train more comfortably for a longer duration. The calculations below will enable you to calculate your ideal training sensitive zone of between 70 and 85 percent of your predicted maximum heart rate. As a general rule, the slower you run, the more likely you are to burn more fat as a preferred source of fuel. Conversely, the faster you run, the more you will rely on carbohydrate as the primary source of fuel.

To measure the intensity at which you are training and to determine whether or not you are running at your desired pace within your training sensitive zone, you'll need to once again measure your heart rate. Follow the instructions below to calculate your training intensity and aerobic training sensitive zone.

Finding Your Aerobic Training Sensitive Zone:

To determine your *predicted maximal heart rate* (PMHR), simply complete the following equation.

Equation: 220 – (your current age) = PMHR

220 - (_____________) = _______beats/minute

Be aware that although the following equation is commonly used, it may overestimate or underestimate predicted maximal heart rate by as much as 15–20 beats.

To calculate your aerobic exercise *training sensitive zone*, simply complete the chart on page 59.

TRAINING SENSITIVE ZONE AND 10-SECOND PULSE COUNT		
A.	220	
B.	(-)	Your age
C.	(=)	Your age predicted maximal heart rate
D.	(x) 0.7	
E.	(=)	The lower limit of your aerobic Training Sensitive Zone
F.	(÷) 6.0	
G.	(=)	Lower limit 10-second pulse count
H.		Your age predicted maximal heart rate
I.	(x) 0.85	
J.	(=)	The upper limit of your aerobic Training Sensitive Zone
K.	(÷) 6.0	
L.	(=)	Upper limit 10-second pulse count

To exercise within your aerobic Training Sensitive Zone, you should exercise at a heart rate of between (E) _______ and (J) _______ beats per minute, or within the 10-second pulse count of (G) _______ and (L) _______ beats.

Another easy way to check the intensity of your pace and confirm that you're not running too fast on a long-distance run is to see if you can hold an effortless conversation with your running partner. If you're able to freely converse, then you are said to be running at a "conversational pace" and you should be fine for completing the distance. Conversely, a very good way to terminate a particularly boring conversation with a running partner is to imperceptively increase the running pace. This may sound a little mean, but when you get to the point where you are logging a lot of miles and running with a wide variety of people, it may prove to be an invaluable strategy.

and if you want to run long you have to learn to run slow." Sounds a little funky, right? Well, it's true. The key to running longer is learning to hold yourself back and running at a much slower pace. This is especially true with long workouts and races. Once you learn to run at a slower pace, you'll be surprised at how much easier and enjoyable it is to run, and how much farther you can go before you fatigue. This is the real-life version of the tortoise and the hare. Be the tortoise.

Running at a slower pace, your muscles will receive sufficient oxygen to break down carbohydrate without producing much lactic acid, and burn more fat as a primary source of fuel. That's an absolute win-win situation. So remember, in terms of increasing the duration of your aerobic training efforts, slow is the way to go.

Training Intensity: After you've been training consistently for a while and have gradually increased the duration of your daily workouts and weekly duration totals, the next progressive step would be to elevate the intensity of your training efforts. This can be achieved by changing your training speed or terrain. If used properly, variations of high-intensity training can have a pronounced effect on your training development and performance. However, "speed kills," so beware, for as good as a little speed training can be, too much is definitely destructive. High-intensity training places tremendous stress on your muscles, tendons, ligaments and bones, so you must be very careful not to overdo it.

To safely and effectively obtain desirable aerobic training health and performance benefits, you should exercise at a pace that produces a heart rate which falls within your calculated training sensitive zone. Using the following information, you can determine which specific training intensity best suits your needs.

High-Intensity Training: If you have established a strong aerobic training foundation and wish to take your training and physical perform-

PACING TABLE		
Target Heart Rate Zone (THRZ)	Training Adaptations	% of maximum
Low Long slow distance (LSD) runs, walks, light jogs	• Improved cardiac and lung efficiency • Increased fat metabolism	60–70%
Moderate Comfortable running, fast-paced walking, stairclimbing (1 step every 2 seconds)	• Highest impact on cardiac and lung capacity/efficiency • Increases number of aerobic organisms in muscle • Greater removal of toxins (lactic acid and carbon dioxide)	70–80%
Moderate-High Short sprints, tempo runs, stairclimbing (1 step every second)	• Improvement of lactate thresholds • Stronger cardiac and lung muscle	80–90%
High Speed/interval training, sprints, power runs, stairclimbing (1 step every .5 seconds)	• Enhanced speed and power of muscle • Should be performed by elite or advanced athletes	90–100%

ance to a higher level, engaging in sessions of higher-intensity training one to three times a week can be very productive. There are a number of different approaches that you can use. The key it to find the one(s) that best fit your needs, desires and abilities. Described below are some successful approaches we have used in the training of our firefighter/athletes. Although the workouts are primarily described in terms of running, the concepts, principles and strategies can all be easily adapted and applied to other forms of aerobic training.

Beginning: One good way to begin increasing the intensity of your workouts is to add a few hills or brief, fast-paced "pick-ups" into the middle of a 30- to 45-minute training effort. Either action will significantly elevate the training stimulus and rapidly promote positive change.

Start out nice and easy and continue at a comfortable pace for at least 10–15 minutes. This should warm up your body and get it ready to go. Now you can either progress through a series of hills or pick up your pace and run a few brief, moderately paced intervals. Take it easy coming down the hills and run at a very conservative pace following your pick-ups so that your body can adequately recover from the intervals of high-intensity work. Once you're sufficiently recovered and feeling good again, give it another shot; take on another hill or run another pick-up. After the completion of a few high-intensity intervals, you should close out your session by exercising at a very comfortable pace for an additional 10–15 minutes.

In your first few sessions, it is particularly important not to overdo it. Take it easy going into the hills and keep your pick-up pace modest; otherwise, you're likely to develop shin splints and injure your Achilles tendon, calf muscles, hamstrings or groin.

Tempo Runs: The most popular type of high-intensity workout is probably the tempo run. With this type of workout, you begin at a comfortable pace and continue for a brief period of time or distance to warm up. Then you switch gears and accelerate to a fairly swift and consistent pace that you can hold for the duration of your run. Another option is to gradually and progressively increase your pace from moderate to high-intensity as you progress through the run. The main objective is to complete the session distance swiftly and to challenge yourself with near-maximal effort.

Interval workouts: Formal interval training is arguably the most painful, productive and potentially destructive method of high-intensity training. If applied to your training program and executed properly, it can produce dramatic improvements in capacity and performance; however, if utilized incorrectly it will destroy you. This level of training should only be attempted by aerobic athletes who already possess a solid foundation of training and are fairly well conditioned. To obtain the greatest benefits from this excellent form of conditioning, you'll need to train with its use on a regular basis, stretch before and after each session, consume a nutritious diet, stay well hydrated and maintain a training balance that provides adequate rest for recovery and development.

In general, the speed workouts we recommend using are about eight to nine miles in length and involve three miles of high-intensity (fast-paced) running intervals. This means that if you're running quarters (400 meters), you should do twelve, with halves (800 meters) you should do six, with 1200 meters you should do four, and with miles (or 1500 meters) you should run three. All workouts should begin with a session of stretching and at least two miles of slow-paced jogging as a warm-up. The high-intensity work should be completed during the middle of the workout and the session should then be closed out with a two-or-so mile light jog for a cool-down.

It's also a good idea to throw in a couple of very brief "striders" (faster-paced running with naturally longer strides) into the second mile of the warm-up. This will fire up all the different muscle fibers involved in the faster-paced movement and stretch out (open up) your running stride. If you elect to toss in a few striders, just don't overdo it; producing and accumulating lactic acid unnecessarily in your warm-up is counterproductive.

Start your intervals just as you would a race—go out pretty quick, accelerating through the first 8-12 strides. Then, upon achieving your desired pace, settle down and concentrate on the maintenance of good running form and steady rhythm. Try to run at an even pace throughout the entire length of the interval. Check your (run-time) splits every 200 meters and immediately adjust your pace as necessary. Running at an even pace throughout the full term of the interval is productive in many ways. Race-pace intervals in particular condition the muscle tissue to operate at an optimal level of efficiency, firing the precise number of fibers necessary to produce the ideal amount of force to propel you forward at the desired rate of speed. Fatigue-producing lactic acid production is also minimized and a clear sense of proper running pace, rhythm and stride is developed.

As you continue to run, lactic acid will progressively accumulate and ultimately cause your muscles to fatigue. In this type of workout, the accumulation of lactic acid rather than the depletion of fuel limits performance. Once you have completed your high-intensity interval, slow your pace to a jog. Jogging slowly will help to remove accumulated lactic acid from the exercised muscles and thereby facilitate recovery. As you near the completion of your recovery interval, your breathing should be normalized and lactic acid levels lowered, but still somewhat higher than normal.

Run each additional high-intensity interval in the same manner as the first. Concentrate on maintaining a proper running pace and good form. Stay mentally focused; the pain and nausea that accompany fatigue will act as a powerful distraction. With each ensuing interval, the initial and final levels of accumulated lactic acid will be progressively higher. As a result, discomfort, pain, nausea and fatigue will occur sooner and become more pronounced. The challenge of these workouts is to win the internal argument of whether to keep going, slow down or stop. It mimics the experience of racing and firefighting. The extremely high levels of lactic acid that are achieved through this specialized method of training inspire the peak development of muscle fiber and mental toughness, both of which are keys to performance at the highest level in the firefield and in the field of athletic competition.

After completing your final high-intensity interval, slow your pace to a comfortable jog and complete at least two miles. Then stretch out lightly, rehydrate and hit the showers.

The following are descriptions of a few classic interval workouts for runners. It's essential that you be in excellent health and very well conditioned to use them. Always exercise lightly or rest on the days which lead up to and follow each interval training session. The total mileage for workouts varies from 7.5 to approximately 10 miles. The most rigorous of the sessions is the Ladder workout. In this workout, you attempt to maintain the same pace with each fast-paced interval as you progressively increase and then decrease the interval distance. The speed intervals in the Mile Repeats B and Ladder Workout should be run at a projected 10-kilometer race pace, the Mile Repeats A at a 5-mile race pace, Mile Repeat C at a 4-mile race pace and the 1200 Meter Repeats at a 5-kilometer race pace.

5. Practice balanced training.

As previously stated, in order to realize the greatest returns from your high-intensity training, you must grant your body sufficient time to rebuild and otherwise positively adapt to the imposed exercise stresses. This is why even the best-trained athletes limit their high-intensity training sessions to just two or three per week. If you get carried away with yourself and compound the exercise stress by training very hard too often, you are going to *blow up*. The productive stress that you impose upon your body will become excessive and result in physical injury; muscle strain, tendon or ligament sprain or shin splints. Train smart and get the most out of your efforts and sacrifices by maintaining a good balance between high-, moderate- and low-intensity training sessions. Always balance long and intense workouts with one or two days of shorter and/or less-intense training sessions.

6. Conduct assessments.

Measuring your initial performance capacity is essential to the development of an "intelligent training program." The results of a good initial pretest will tell you exactly where you are and thereby

	Warm-up	Speed Interval	Reps	Recovery Interval	Cool Down	Miles
Mile Repeats A	2 miles	1 mile	3	½ mile (800 m)	2 miles	8
Mile Repeats B	2 miles	1 mile	4	½ mile (800 m)	2 miles	9.5
Mile Repeats C	2 miles	1 mile	3	¼ mile (400 m)	2 miles	7.5
1200-Meter Repeats	2 miles	1200 meters	4	400 meters	2 miles	7.75
800-Meter Repeats	2 miles	800 meters	6	400 meters	2 miles	8.25
400-Meter Repeats	2 miles	400 meters	12	200 meters	2 miles	8.5
Ladder Workout	2 miles	400 meters	1	200 meters	2 miles	9.87
		800 meters	1	400 meters		
		1200 meters	1	600 meters		
		1 mile	1	800 meters		
		1200 meters	1	600 meters		
		800 meters	1	400 meters		
		400 meters	1			

provide you with a clearer picture of how to begin and how far you have to go to achieve your training goal(s). In knowing the start and end-points of your training program, you are clearly in the best position to develop a more realistic and effective "personalized" training program.

The fundamental test that we used to determine the aerobic fitness levels of FDNY Academy firefighters was the 1.5-mile run. We simply timed the firefighters' run at the onset of their training and then placed them into performance-based groups for their training runs. Training in ability-based groups facilitated their rate of development. You should operate in a similar manner. Conduct your own personal pre-test with whatever form of aerobic exercise you decide to use. Then knowing where you are and where you want to go, construct your personal training schedule, gradually increasing your frequency, duration and intensity as previously described. Once you have been training successfully for some time, a particularly rewarding way to assess your current level of aerobic fitness and training progress is through participation in athletic competition. If your aerobic training involves either running, swimming or cycling, you should consider participating in a local race. In terms of selecting a successful race pace, a good friend once advised me that "if you don't go out fast, you'll never run your *best* race"[10]. He was right, as it related to the high-end level of competition that we were competing at during that time. However, as a general rule and especially at the beginning and novice levels, you should always run smart first, and then run tough. Go out conservatively, and then build to a strong and successful finish. The runners I knew who trained and raced smart enjoyed great success, feasting on those who tragically went out too fast and consequently crashed and burned. Again, if you run smart from the start, you'll run strong to the end. That's the way to achieve peak performance.

7. Warm up and cool down.

Always begin and complete your aerobic training sessions with a comfortably paced warm-up and cool-down. Most runners complete these essential tasks by stretching and then jogging at a very light pace. Stretching and otherwise warming up your muscles prior to a run improves training performance while minimizing the potential for injury. Two additional thoughts in regards to pre-session stretching are: a) the more intense the workout, the more important it is to stretch and b) the older you get the more apparent this becomes.

The idea of a cool-down is to facilitate recovery by washing out the unwanted by-products of exercise stress from your muscles, to supply fresh nutrients to the exercised tissues and to return the status of your muscles to a more loosened and relaxed state. The 10–15 minutes that you invest in your warm-up and cool-down are likely to produce extremely valuable returns. After completing a race or high-intensity workout, be sure to always stretch slowly, comfortably and comprehensively.

Strength Training

Firefighting is a physically demanding total body activity. Working in heavy and restrictive protective clothing and performing strenuous tasks in punishing environments, firefighters must possess great total body strength and muscular endurance. To develop these capacities, firefighters need to train consistently, intensely and comprehensively. Circuit-type resistance training provides the specific type of training stimulus necessary to meet the unique strength conditioning needs of firefighters. It presents a rigorous total body muscular challenge that mimics occupational demands, thereby facilitating the development of important body-wide and cellular-level muscle fibers changes. Training with the use of the following circuit-type resistance training programs will aid you in increasing total body muscular endurance and strength. Within weeks you are going to look better, feel better and perform at a significantly higher level. Continued work will enable you to achieve the much greater goal of attaining the peak level of fitness importantly possessed and routinely displayed by high-intensity, high-performance firefighters.

In the 1970s, a New York City firefighter named James Myerjack developed a circuit-type resistance training program that was specifically designed to improve his and other firefighter's performance capacities in the fire field. Jim worked as a firefighter in a very busy ladder company in the South Bronx, Ladder Company 19. He was a huge man (with an even bigger heart), an outstanding firefighter and an accomplished power lifter—the kind of firefighter who you'd expect could pull the door off its hinges just as soon as force it open with the use of tools. Interestingly, however, at a point in his career, Jim was stated to have been disappointed with his personal firefighting performance. He claimed to notice that "men half his size could physically outperform him on the fireground."[12] Looking at Jim, and knowing of his incredible reputation as a firefighter, you couldn't help but think that his personal assessment may have been a tad overstated. Nevertheless, Jim was quite serious about wanting to improve his personal firefighting capacities, so he combined his knowledge of firefighting and resistance training to create an original resistance-training program. Jim's program has been a tremendous success, being used by the FDNY Health & Fitness Unit to improve the health, safety and performance capacities of more than 20,000 FDNY members over the past 25 years. Similar programs have been developed and successfully employed by other knowledgeable firefighters in progressive departments such as Deputy Chief Scott Peltin (retired) with the Phoenix Fire Department in Arizona.

Jim's intention was to develop a strength-training program that would enable him and other firefighters to successfully contend with the genuine physical challenges of the fire field. These included such feats as forcing open numerous doors, overhauling the entire ceiling of a room or extinguishing several rooms of fire. Recognizing the need for muscular endurance and total body development, he divided the body into 11 different areas and utilized exercises to develop the muscles in each of these regions. He also prescribed the completion of many (25–30) repetitions for first-set exercises, the use of short recovery periods, slow eccentric movements (where the active muscles are lengthened), relatively light weights and the gradual building from one to three exercise sets.

Our series of programs are an extension of Jim's work. Emphasizing the primary concepts of total body conditioning and the development of muscular endurance, we have created several unique and exciting training programs. In an effort to provide motivating training options and to afford you the luxury of conditioning at almost anytime and anywhere, we have also provided both gym and home versions of each program using a variety of resistance equipment, free weights and calisthenic exercises. Hopefully these options will make it easier for you to train more frequently and optimize the rate of your development. Finally, to help you understand the direct connect that exists between our prescribed training exercises and genuine firefighting tasks, we have provided photographically supported written descriptions of the relationships that exists between each exercise and its coupled firefighting task.

With all four primary programs, moderate resistance is combined with the completion of 15–20 (or more) repetitions, and 10 or 12 exercises to develop all the body's major muscle groups. Resistance exercises are completed in a deliberate manner, featuring two distinct movements designed to maximize development. The initial concentric action (where the active muscles are shortened) is completed swiftly and powerfully in 1–2 seconds time, while the second eccentric movement (where the active muscle is lengthened) is done more slowly in 3–4 seconds. By design, the rapid concentric movement effectively simulates firefighting muscle action and encourages the development of muscular strength and power. The slower, more controlled eccentric movement inspires changes that help to improve muscular strength and endurance.

Strong emphasis is also placed on the concept of *continuous motion*. This is done to simulate the muscle activity involved with real firefighting actions, to encourage the development of muscular endurance and to gain some aerobic training effect. Exercise repetitions of 15 to 20 (or more) are completed in a continuous manner through a period of approximately 45–60 seconds. Each exercise is then followed by a brief period (15–30 seconds) of recovery, as one rapidly moves to and then makes any necessary adjustments to equipment at the next exercise station. The combination of high repetitions, brief recovery, total body involvement and multiple sets produces elevated levels of lactic acid. This stimulates positive muscle development and a heart rate response that generally falls within the lower end of the aerobic training sensitive zone. Working continuously at this level of intensity for 20 or more minutes is likely to inspire cardiovascular (aerobic) training effect.

Two additional benefits to be obtained through the consistent use of these training programs are increases in muscle mass and elevated muscular activity. As a consequence of your efforts, your muscles will become larger, more defined and more active. This is very useful if you're trying to increase muscular stature and simultaneously lose some body fat. Muscle, unlike fat, is always very active, even at rest. It requires a great deal of energy to maintain a constant state of readiness to perform. Therefore, the more developed your muscles become as a result of training, the more calories they will burn *all the time*. The bottom line is that by consistently training with the use of these programs, not only will you become bigger, stronger and better defined, but you'll also develop into a virtual metabolic machine.

This training methodology, the programs and their exercises are all especially designed to optimize the rate of training gains and performance capacities of firefighters, as well as current and aspiring athletes. Your consistent training with the use of these programs will therefore generate strength and muscular endurance improvements that will enable you to excel in the athletic field and look, feel and perform on the level of a high-intensity firefighter. Moreover, for current and prospective firefighters, routine and progressive conditioning with the use of these programs can increase engine company or ladder company firefighting ability. Firefighter candidates will also be well served through the use of these programs. Their training investments can translate directly into the earning of a professional firefighting career.

Training Benefits

Consistent training with the use of these strength-conditioning programs will produce many additional health and performance-oriented benefits. The following are some of the more important positive changes:

- Increases the efficiency of the nervous system and muscle fibers to produce a more coordinated and forceful muscle contraction, and increases the number of special intramuscular proteins responsible for generating a more forceful contraction.
- Increases your ability to take in, transport, deliver and utilize oxygen to produce energy for continued muscle contraction(s).
- Increases the concentration of enzymes in the muscle cell responsible for producing energy without the use of oxygen (anaerobically) and improves the ability to break down carbohydrate in the muscle cell so that it can be used as a fuel source for muscle energy production.
- Increases the number of high-energy storing molecules within the muscle fiber.
- Increases your ability to dispose and tolerate higher levels of fatigue-causing lactic acid.
- Increases the strength of your tendons (which connect muscle to bone) and ligaments (which connect bone to bone) to increase the stability of your joints and assist with forceful muscle contractions.
- Increases the amount of calories your muscle burns at rest and during exercise.
- Decreases the amount of excess, unwanted and unhealthy body fat.
- Improves your ability to move sugar from your blood to your muscle.
- Improves your ability to move more quickly, safely and powerfully.

General Strength-Training Protocol

The following guidelines are specifically designed for use with the Firefighter I Workout but may also be applied to any of the other programs presented here.

1. It is always a good idea to warm up prior to your resistance training session with a comprehensive

set of static stretching exercises and 5–10 minutes of low-intensity aerobic exercise (walking, slow jogging, cycling, etc.). Warming up and stretching your muscular and connective tissues prior to training will have an undeniably positive effect on your workout. A good general body warm-up increases circulation and elevates body temperature in a positive way. It also improves oxygen and nutrient delivery to working muscles and increases the activity of energy-producing enzymes. Even a minor (1°C) rise in muscle tissue temperature produces dramatic increases in muscle enzyme activity. This is, of course, the literal reason for "warming up" prior to participation in vigorous forms of activity.

We recommend that you complete the full Firefighter I Flexibility program (page 40) prior to beginning your resistance-training session. Completing this comprehensive set of stretching exercises will help you to move with greater ease, thereby increasing the efficiency, safety and effectiveness of your exercise movements.

2. If you're relatively new to this type of activity, it is highly recommended that you begin your strength training with the use of resistance equipment as opposed to free weights. Training with resistance equipment is very safe and facilitates the development of balanced and coordinated lifting movements.

   Once you've developed your lifting technique and skills, you can switch to free weights (dumbbells and barbells). Free weights and cable machines should be your ultimate choice for training if you desire to maximize your lifting gains and optimize the degree of transfer from training to field performance. Using these training tools, you can modify exercise movements to very closely match athletic or firefighting actions. Muscles that stabilize the body during the activity, as well as those that support and assist the primary muscle(s) involved with the movement are also developed. This produces much more extensive and complete muscular development.

3. Power into each exercise, and then return smoothly and slowly to the initial position. The powerful concentric movement into the exercise should take between 1–2 seconds. The ("negative") eccentric movement, which returns you to the initial exercise position, should ideally be completed within 3–4 seconds. As they say in the world of resistance training, emphasizing the negative produces very positive results. Eccentric movements are key in facilitating muscle growth and development (hypertrophy). In total, each exercise should take about 45–60 seconds to complete.

4. Focus on taking your movement through the full range of motion. Try to move smoothly, in a very fluid and controlled manner. In Jim's words, "Take [your] body parts to the limit without straining."[12] Never compromise your form in an effort to eke out one last repetition. It's not worth the risk of injury. It's good to train tough, but winners train smart first, then they get tough.

5. BREATHE! Do not hold your breath when lifting. By holding your breath as you exert yourself, you can create some very serious blood pressure issues and consequences. *Exhalation* with *execution* is definitely the way to go. Push the air from your lungs at a constant rate as you power into the dynamic movement.

6. Complete between 15–20 repetitions of each exercise as indicated in the respective program. Once you've completed 20 repetitions at a given resistance for a few sessions, increase the resistance slightly. Don't overdo it with the increases, though, as you're much better off taking small progressive steps. Remember, small steps generally result in the largest gains.
7. Move directly from one exercise to the next. Ideally, you should begin your next exercise within 15 seconds of completing the last. This simulates the *real* physical nature of "the job" and keeps your heart rate elevated to the point where you are likely to gain an aerobic-training effect.
8. Working almost continuously and at a fairly high level of intensity, you'll produce quite a bit of lactic acid and therefore possibly feel a little nauseous during the latter stages of the first few training sessions. This is a normal body response and typically passes after the completion of 2–4 sessions. To minimize this effect, we recommend that you slow things down a little for the first few sessions; proceed through the circuit at a slightly slower rate and take a little more time to recover between each exercise.
9. Upon the completion of your resistance-training program, you should complete a comprehensive set of stretching exercises, emphasizing the muscle groups targeted in your training routine. This should be followed by a low-intensity aerobic cool-down (5 to 10 minutes). These added training components assist in the clearing of lactic acid from your exercised muscles and bloodstream, actively facilitating the recovery of fatigued muscles. Make sure that you grant your body sufficient time to replenish and develop by limiting your total-body workout sessions to a maximum of three per week. Ideally, you should take at least one recovery day following each full training session; for those of you who alternate body regions in your workouts, you should never work the same muscle groups intensely two days in a row. As an example, most of our firefighter/athletes complete full-body circuits on Monday, Wednesday and Friday or Tuesday, Thursday and Saturday.
10. Once you've developed a sound foundation with your strength training, it's a very good idea to vary the exercises of your routine, the intensity and number of exercise repetitions and the planes of exercise movement. This will facilitate continued development (neuromuscular function and hypertrophy), make the workouts more interesting and help you to avoid staleness or plateauing.

Four principle and three alternative strength-training programs have been provided to meet your specific conditioning needs or interests. Review the program descriptions and select the best-fit program(s) for you. Then just get on out there and do it; enjoy the workouts and relish the gains.

Strength-Training Programs

FIREFIGHTER I WORKOUT

The first program is designed specifically for individuals with little or no previous resistance-training experience. It simultaneously develops lifting techniques and skills, improves capacities and builds a strong resistance-training foundation. It's also a very good program for those interested in attaining and maintaining a rock-solid base of total body fitness. By design, the Firefighter I program is easy to learn and simple to use.

Note: This program presents an array of free-weight exercises as well as their machine counterparts. If you are new to resistance training, we highly recommend that you visit a gym and perform the machine exercises with the guidance of the gym's fitness staff. These machine exercises will help you develop balanced and coordinated lifting movements that are essential for the proper execution of free-weight exercises.

Begin by completing just one set. Once you've gotten used to the training, you should expand your session by adding a second and eventually third full set. We highly recommend that you complete a warm-up composed of light aerobic exercise and stretching prior to your training session. A low-intensity aerobic cool-down combined with some light stretching would be excellent as well.

1. Dumbbell Heel Raise

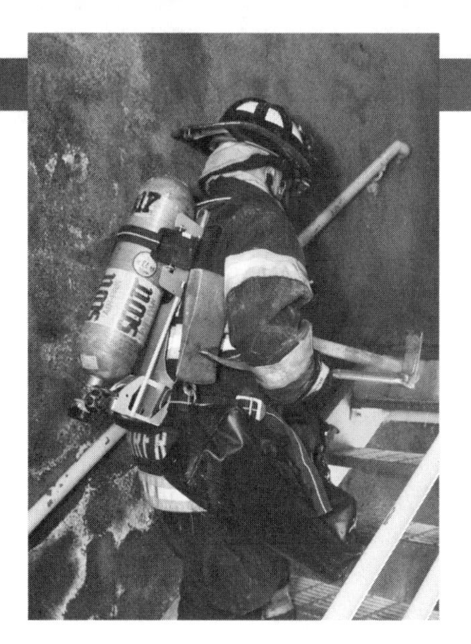

Target: Gastrocnemius

Starting Position: Stand with your feet about shoulder-width apart, holding the hand weights at your sides.

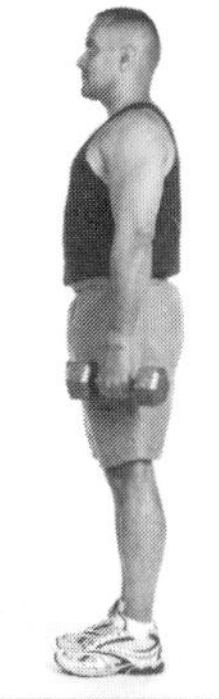

Starting Position

1. Raise your heels up off the ground and pause.
2. Slowly return to starting position.

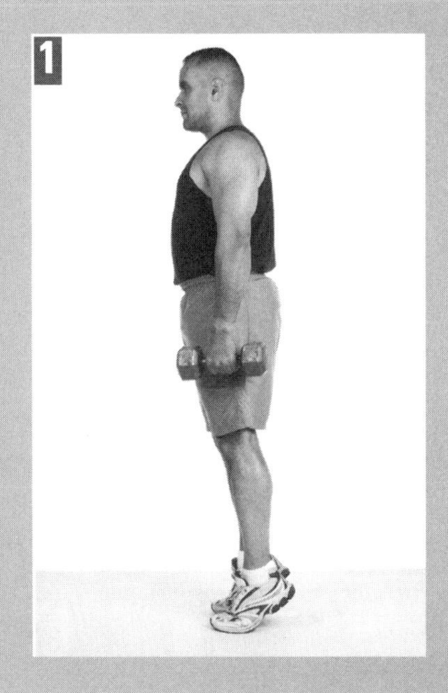

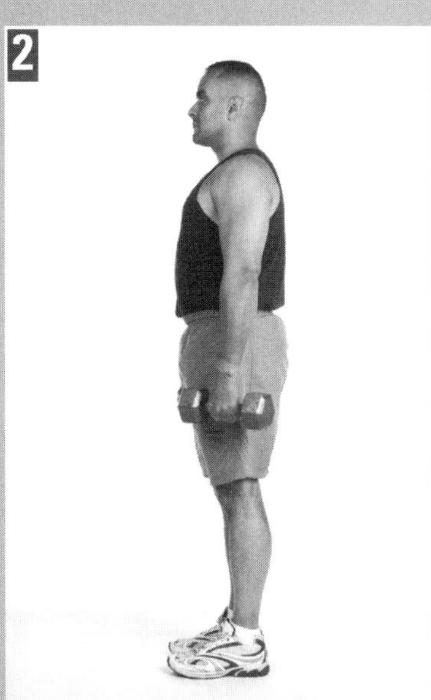

Machine Counterpart: Machine Heel Raise

2. Dumbbell Lunge

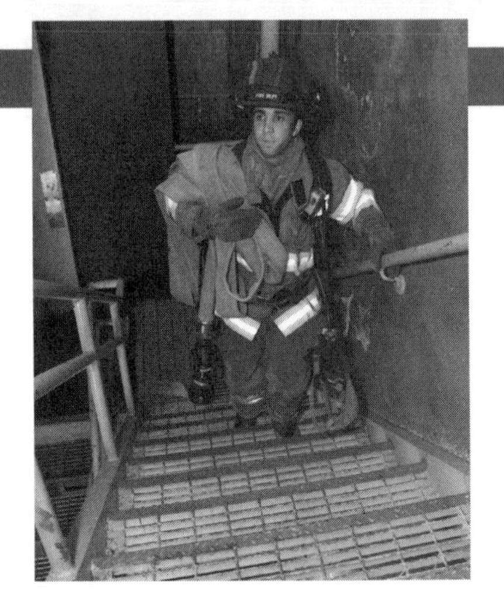

Target: Quadriceps, hamstrings, gastrocnemius

Starting Position: Stand with your feet about shoulder-width apart, holding the hand weights at your sides.

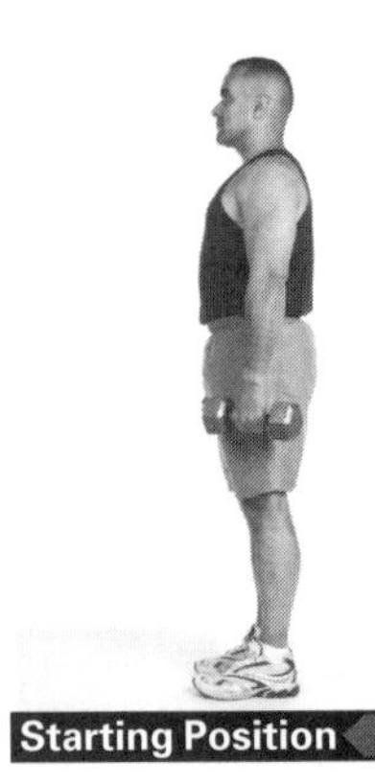

Starting Position

1. Take a large step forward, bend the front leg to about 90 degrees, and pause.
2. Push off the floor with the front leg and return to starting position.

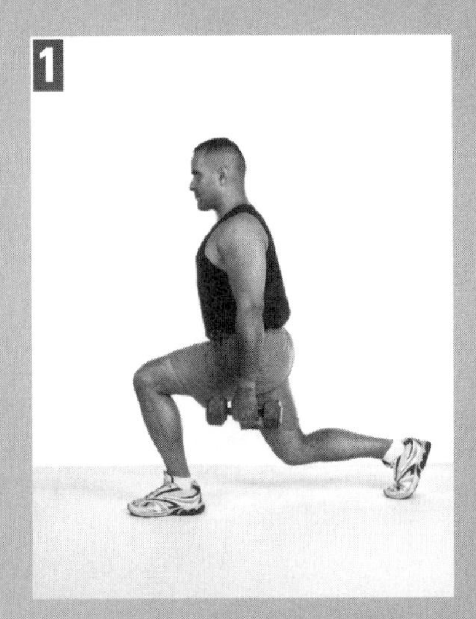

1

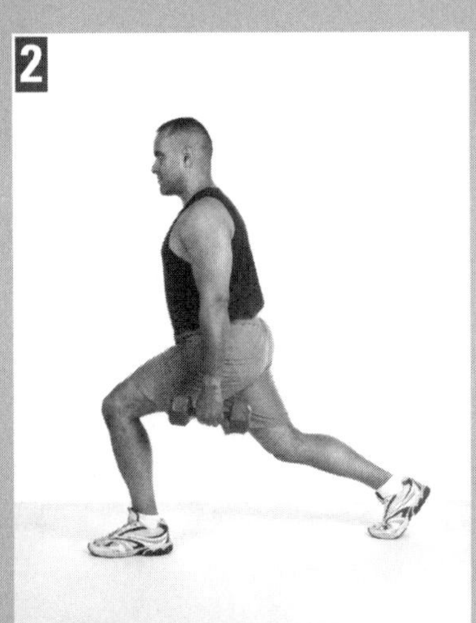

2

Machine Counterpart: Seated Leg Curl

3. Dumbbell Squat

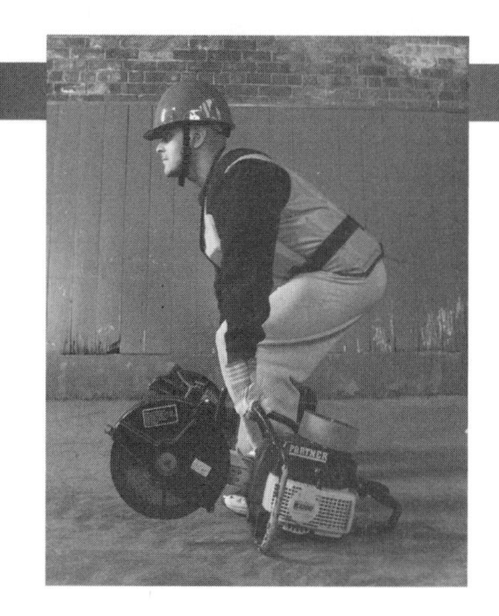

Target: Gastrocnemius, quadriceps

Starting Position: Stand with your feet slightly wider than shoulder-width apart, holding the hand weights at your sides.

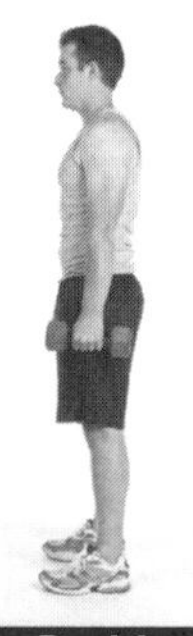

Starting Position

1. Bend your knees, moving into a sitting position, and hold.
2. Slowly return to starting position.

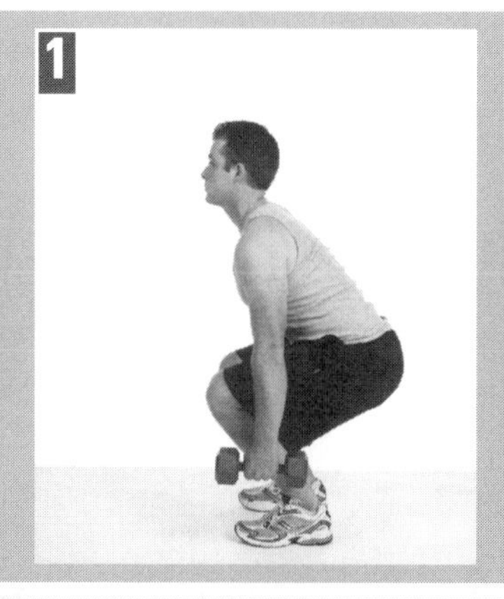

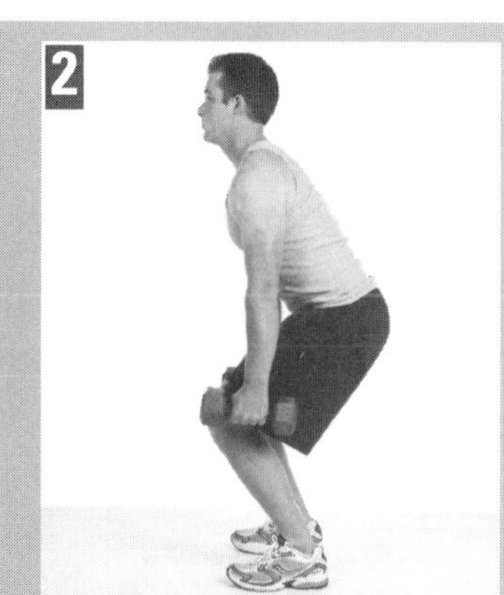

Machine Counterpart: Machine Leg Press

1. Lie down and press your lower back against the support pad. Place your feet about shoulder-width apart on the footplate. Turn the locks out of the way and grasp the handles. Bend your knees toward your chest.
2. Slowly extend your legs. Hold. Slowly return to starting position.

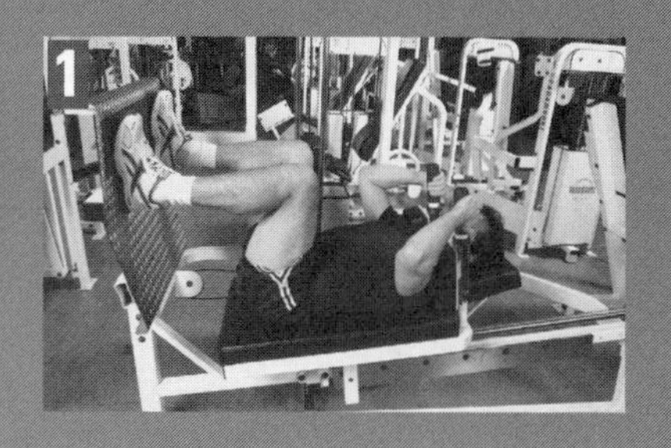

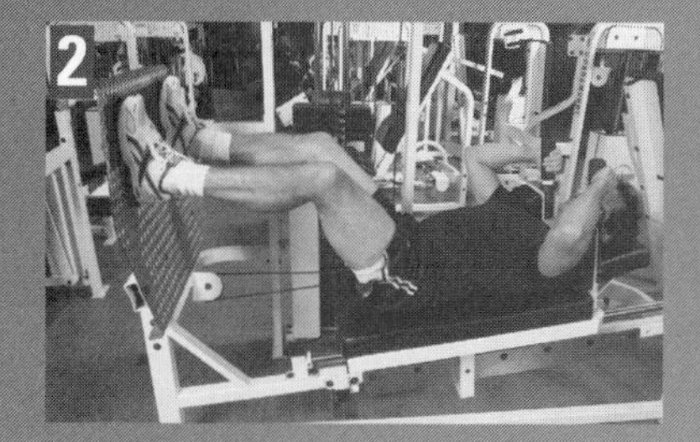

4. Crunch

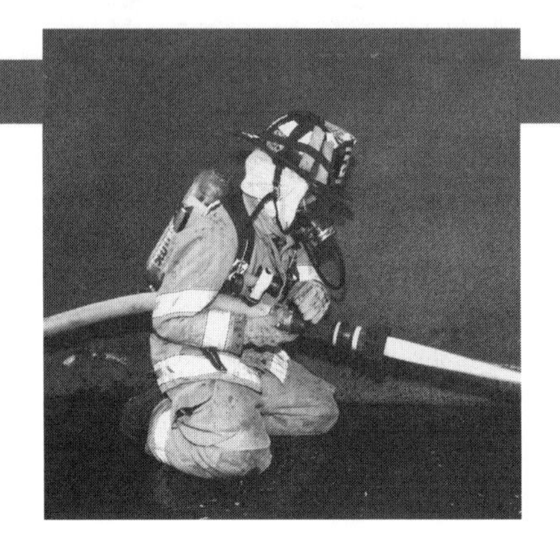

Target: Rectus abdominis

Starting Position: Lie on your back and bend your knees to about 90 degrees, placing your feet flat on the floor. Fold your arms across your chest.

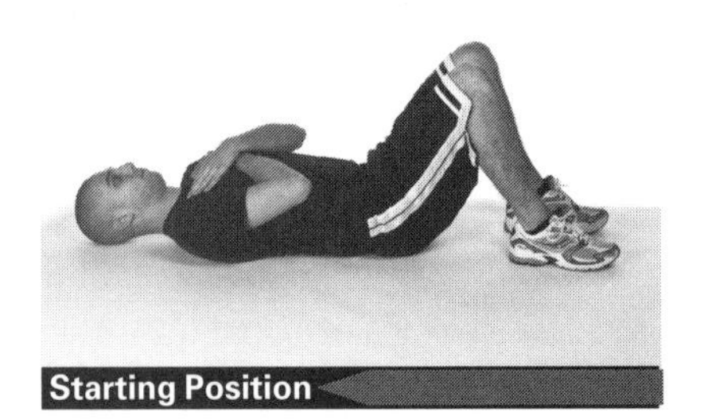
Starting Position

1 Slowly raise your shoulders a few inches off the ground and hold.

2 Slowly return to starting position.

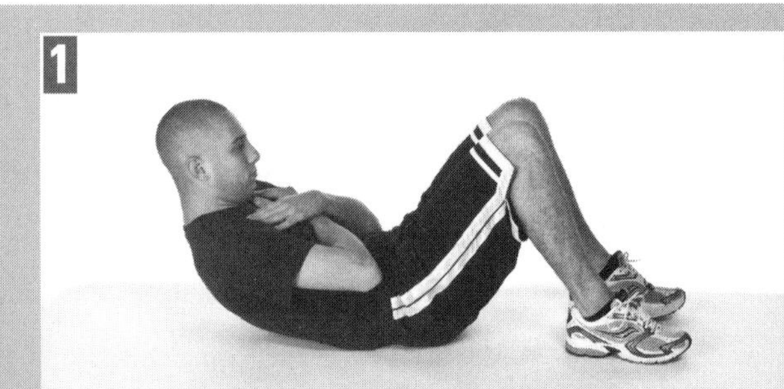

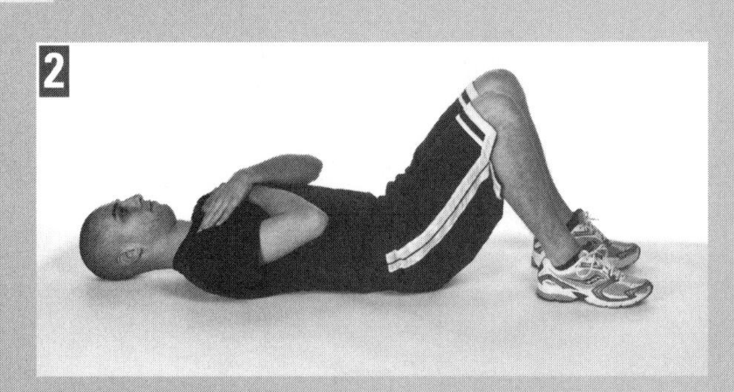

Machine Counterpart: Machine Abdominal Crunch

5. Back Extension

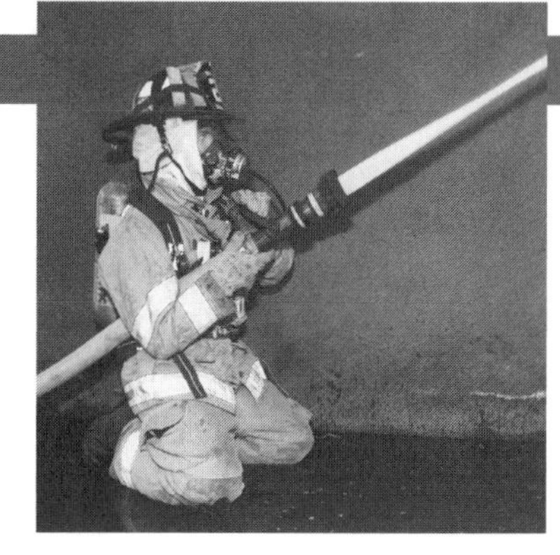

Target: Spinal erectors

Starting Position: Lie face down on the ground. Stack your hands on the floor and rest your chin on them.

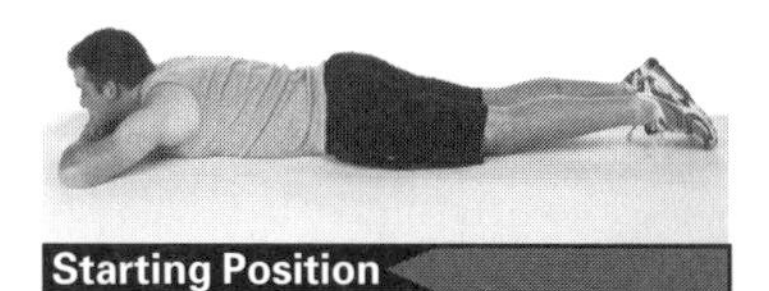

Starting Position

1 Slowly raise your arms and legs off the ground a few inches and hold.

2 Slowly return to starting position.

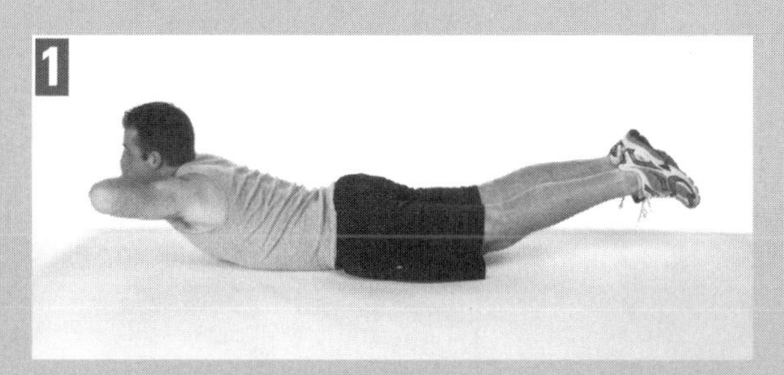

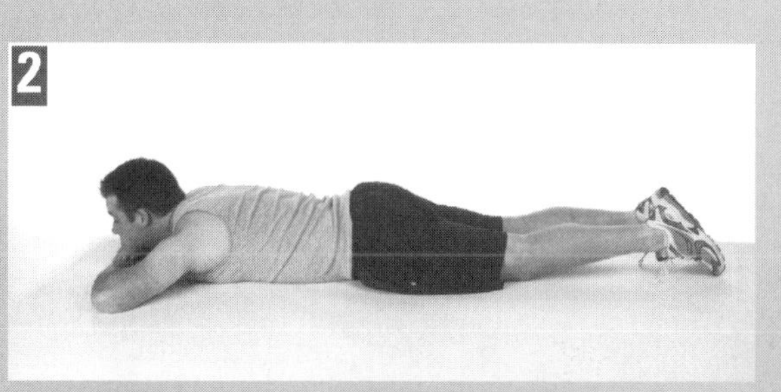

Machine Counterpart: Machine Back Extension

1 Push against the pad until you are reclined. Hold.

2 Slowly return to starting position.

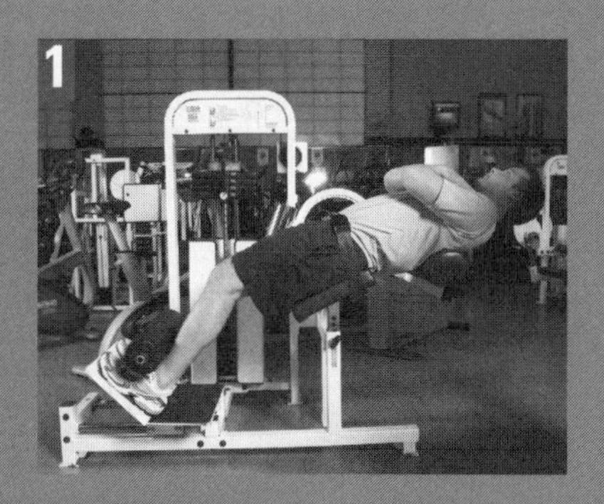

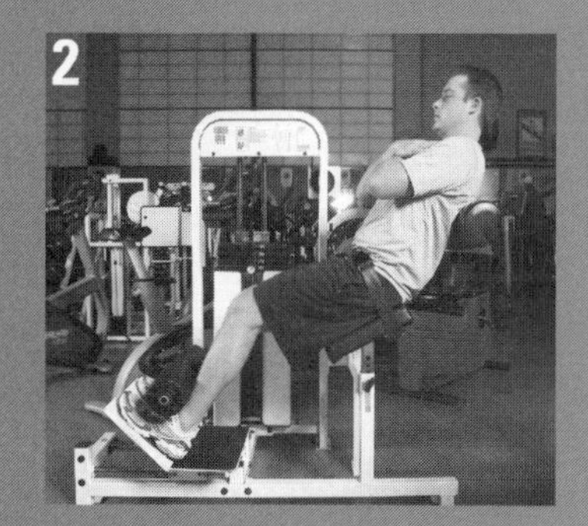

6. Push-Up

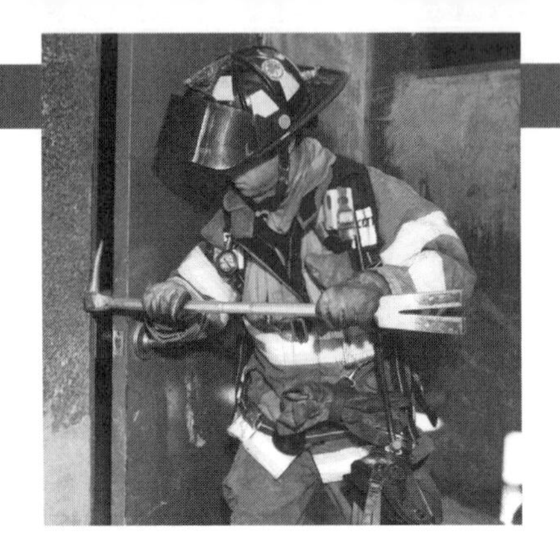

Target: Pectorals

Starting Position: Place your hands slightly wider than shoulder-width apart on the ground. Walk your feet back until your legs are straight and your body forms a straight line from your heels to the top of your head.

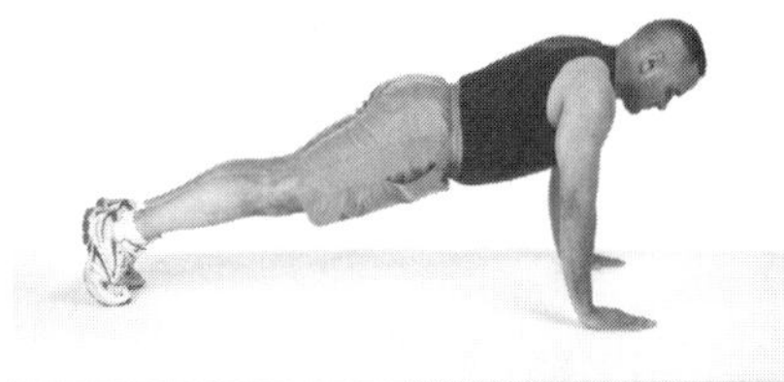

Starting Position

1. Slowly lower down until your chest is one inch from the floor.
2. Press your body up from the floor and hold.

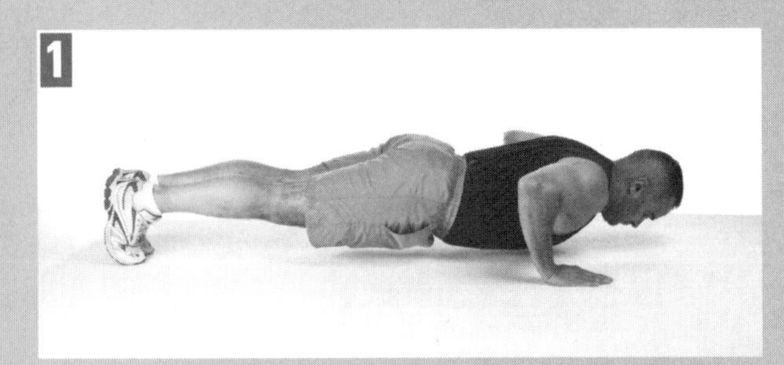

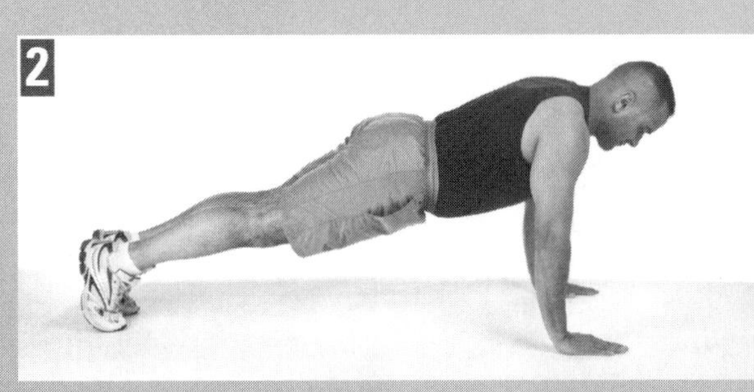

Machine Counterpart: Machine Bench Press

7. Dumbbell One-Arm Row

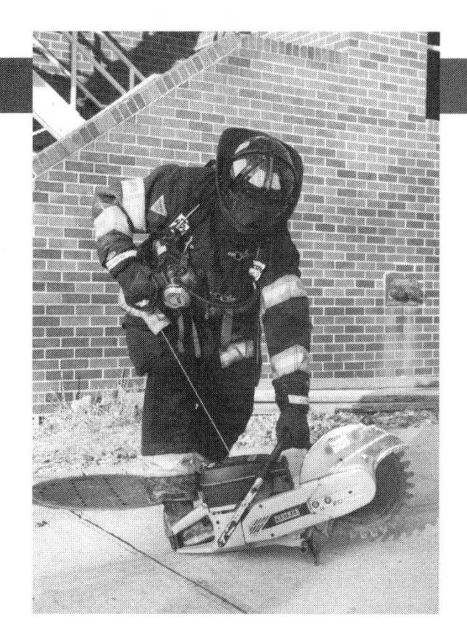

Target: Latissimus dorsi, teres major, posterior deltoid, rhomboids, trapezius, biceps

Starting Position: Bend over and place one hand on a chair. Hold the weight with the other hand and let it hang to the ground. Keep your knees bent and your back straight.

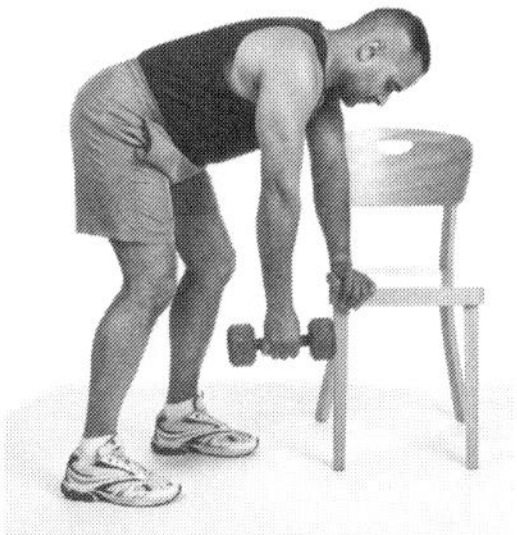

Starting Position

1. Leading with your elbow, lift the weight straight up and hold.
2. Slowly return to starting position.

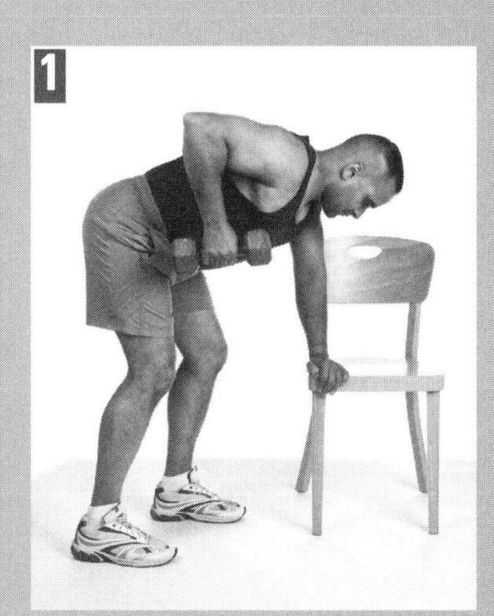

1

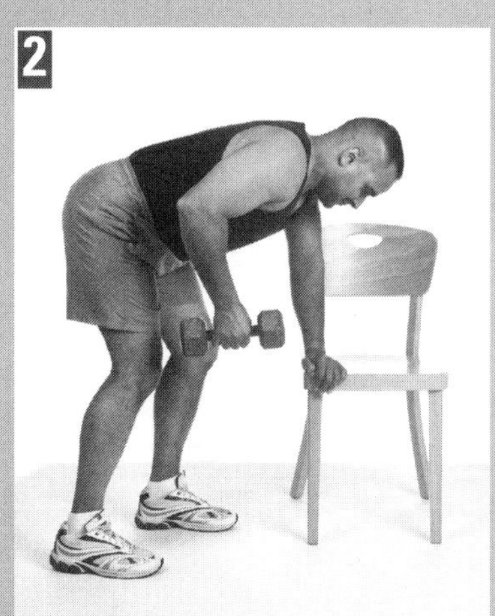

2

Machine Counterpart: Seated Row

8. Dumbbell Overhead Press

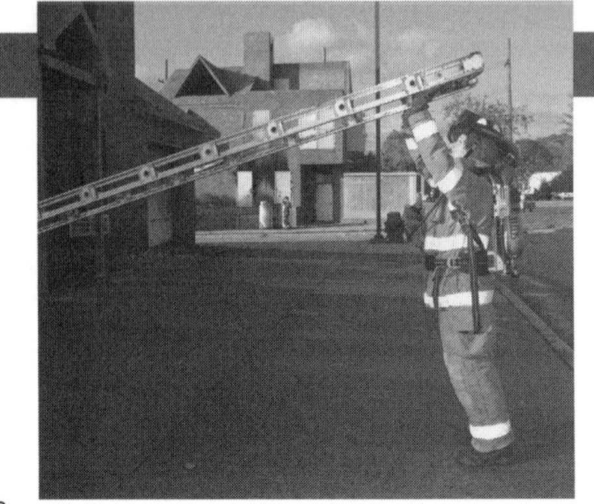

Target: Deltoids, triceps

Starting Position: Stand with your feet about shoulder-width apart, holding the hand weights at shoulder level with your palms facing upward.

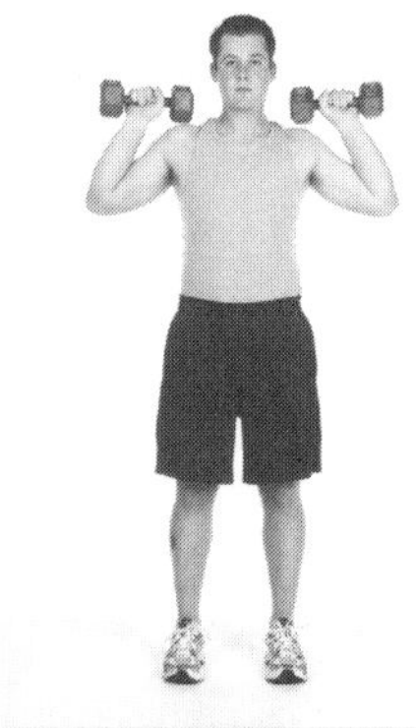

Starting Position

1. Press straight up until your elbows are almost fully extended and hold.
2. Slowly return to starting position.

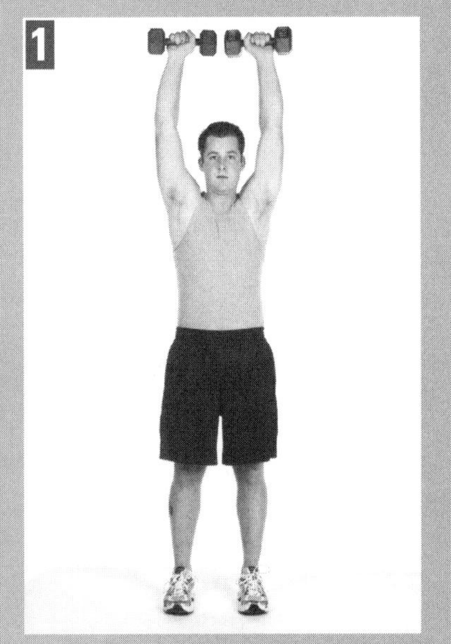

1

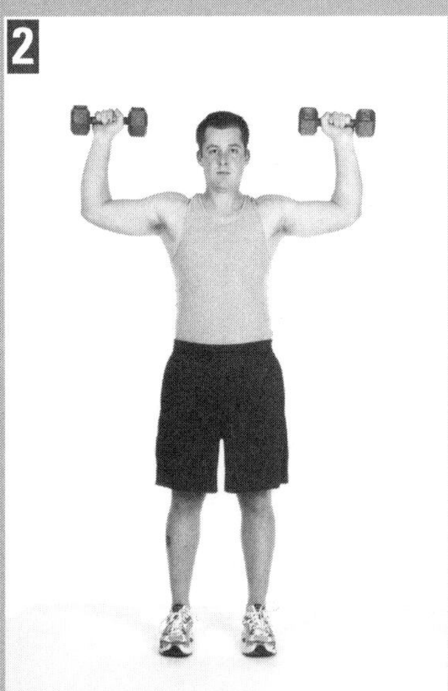

2

Machine Counterpart: Machine Overhead Press

9. Dumbbell Twisting Curl

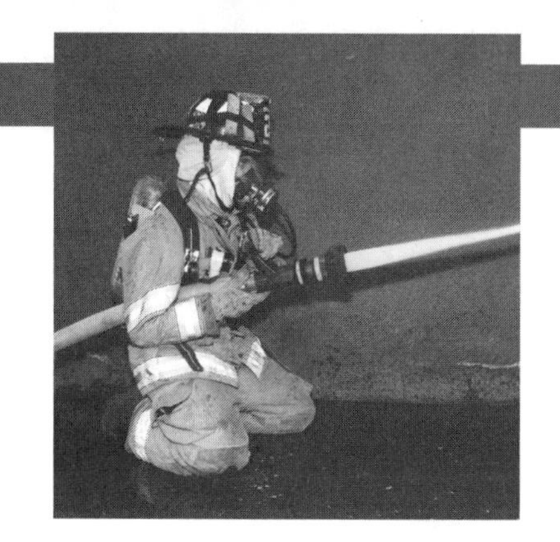

Target: Biceps

Starting Position: Stand with your feet about shoulder-width apart, holding the weights at your sides with your palms facing inward.

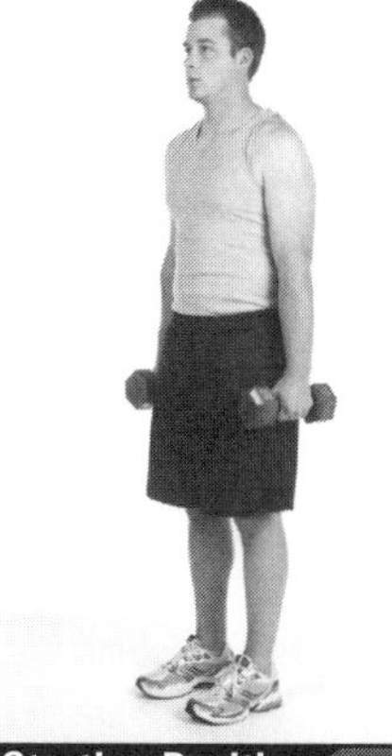

Starting Position

1. Bend your elbows to curl the weights toward your shoulders while twisting your palms to face your body; hold.
2. Slowly return to starting position.

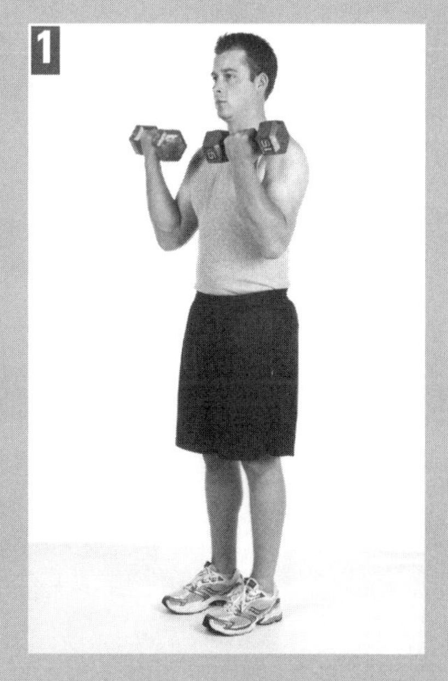

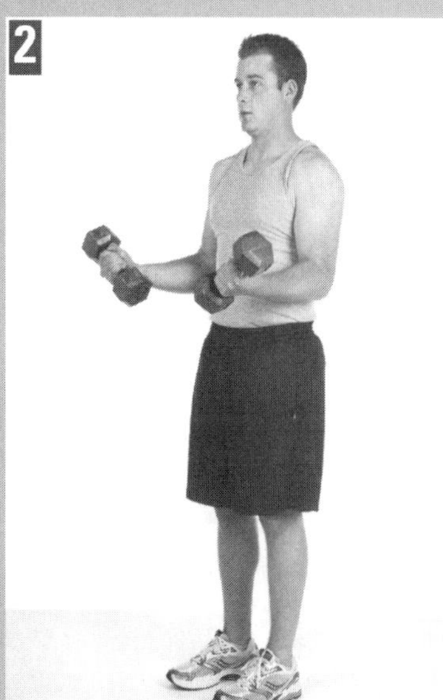

Machine Counterpart: Cable Curl

10. Dumbbell Kickback

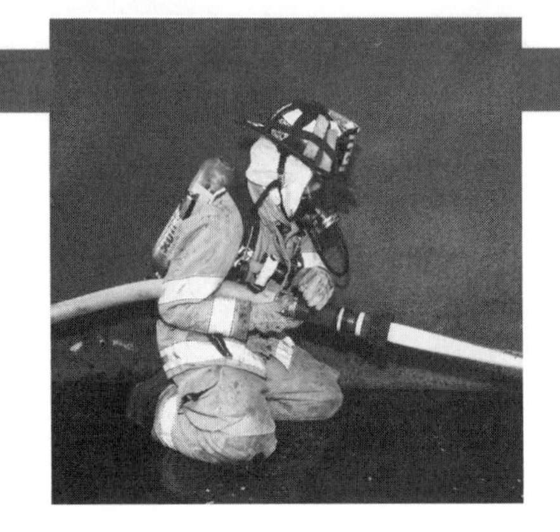

Target: Triceps

Starting Position: Bend over and place one hand on a chair. Hold the dumbbell in the other hand. Your upper arm should be next to your side and your elbow should be bent at a 90-degree angle, with your lower arm directed downward toward the ground.

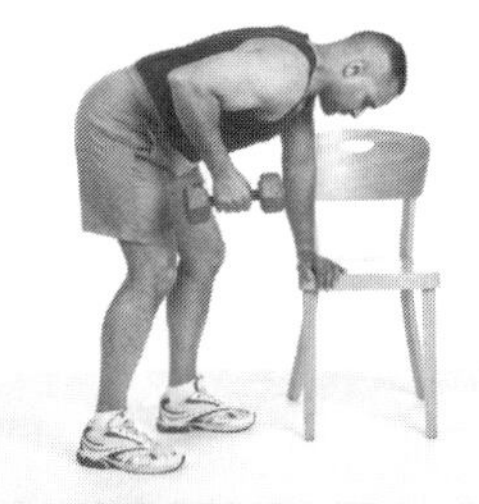

Starting Position

1. Keeping your upper arm next to your side, reach the weight back and straighten your elbow; hold.
2. Slowly return to starting position.

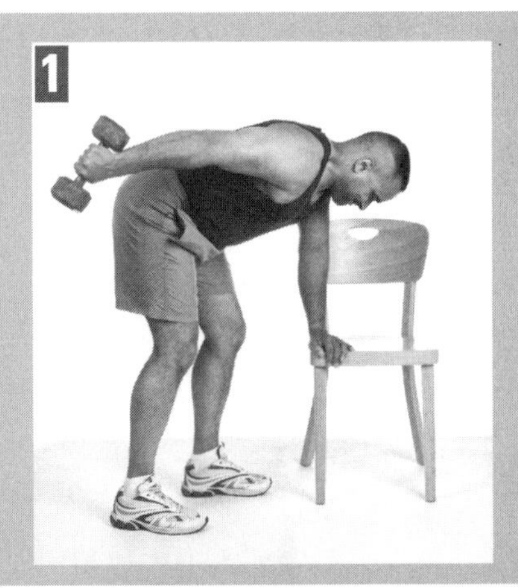

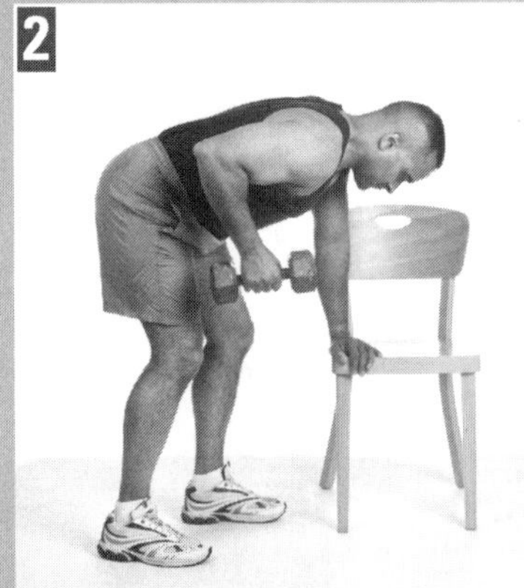

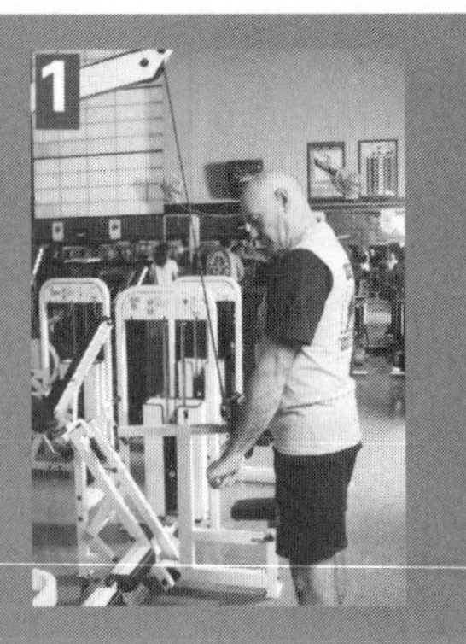

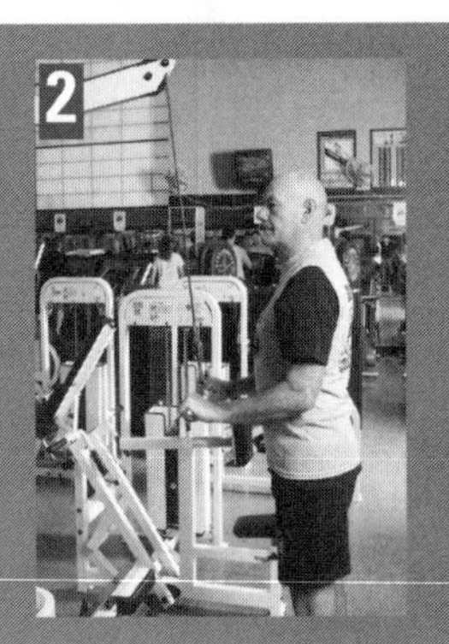

Alternative: Cable Triceps Press-Down

1. Stand with your feet about shoulder-width apart, facing the cable machine. Grasp the bar at chest level and keep your elbows at your sides.
2. Extend your arms downward until they are straight and hold. Slowly return to starting position.

11. Dumbbell Shrug

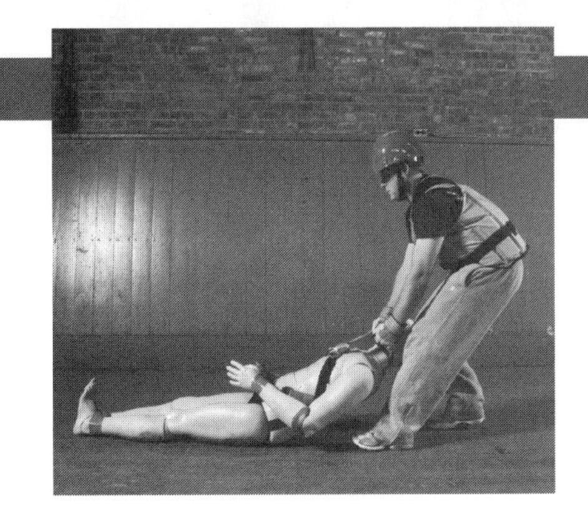

Target: Upper trapezius

Starting Position: Stand with your feet about shoulder-width apart and hold the hand weights in front of your thighs.

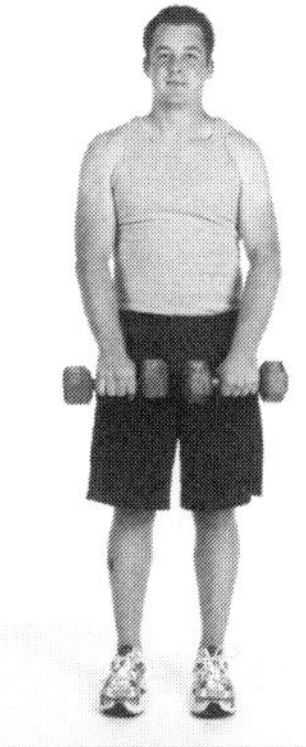

Starting Position

1. Elevate your shoulders toward your ears; hold.
2. Slowly return to starting position.

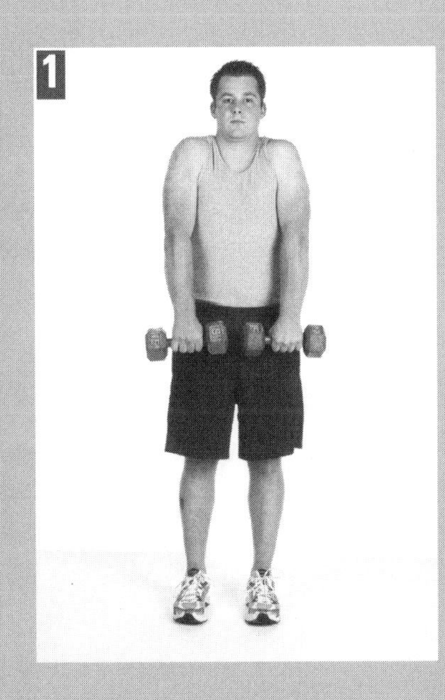

1

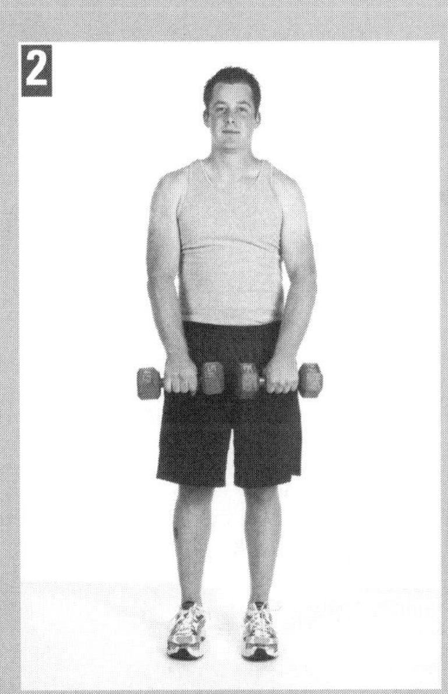

2

Machine Counterpart: Cable Shrug

12. Dumbbell Wrist Roll

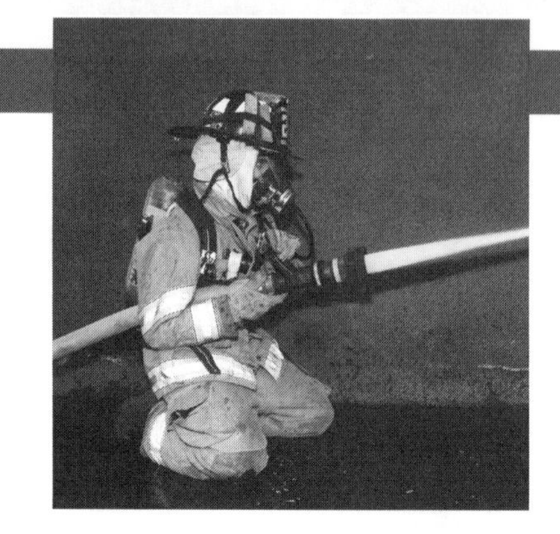

Target: Brachioradialis

Starting Position: Sitting on the edge of a chair or bench, grasp a weight in each hand and place your forearms and elbows on your thighs; your palms should face you. Lean forward.

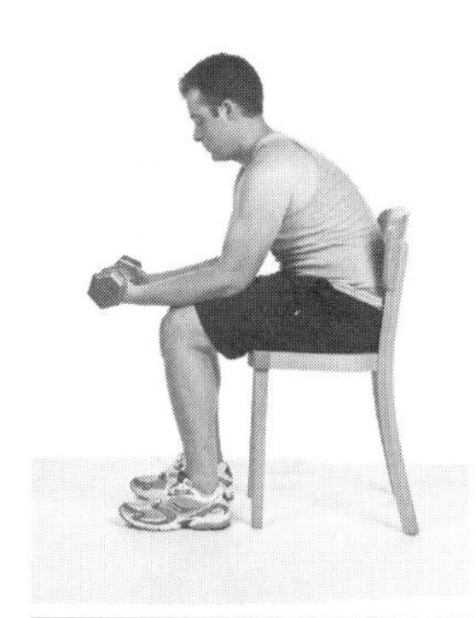

Starting Position

1 Flex your wrists toward the floor.

2 Return to starting position.

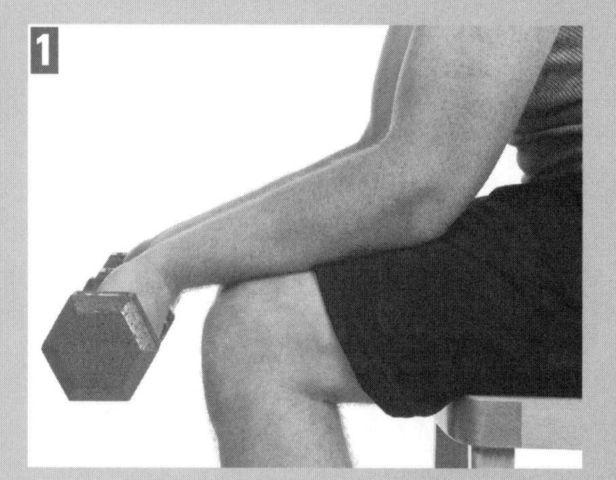

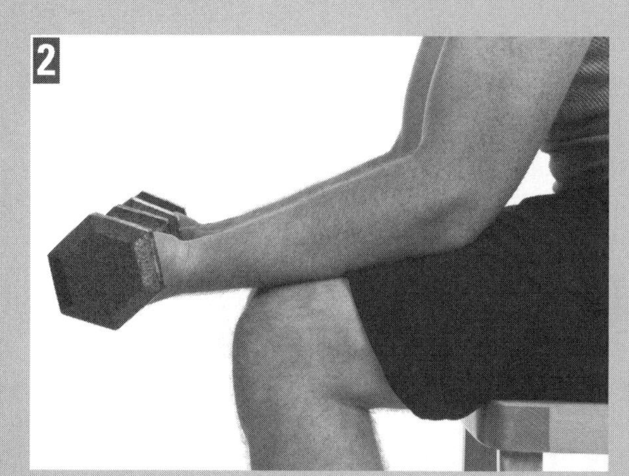

Machine Counterpart: Cable Wrist Roll

ENGINE COMPANY NOZZLEMAN'S WORKOUT

The nozzleman position is *the* position in the fire service. This is the person who literally puts out the fire. The fitness needs of this person cannot be overstated; everyone's life depends on the nozzleman getting the job done. This training program focuses on the development of muscles used extensively by the nozzleman to extinguish fire. It targets muscles in the core, arms and shoulders, with particular emphasis placed on the biceps. This workout is perfect for firefighters who want to be able to extinguish every room of fire they encounter, as well as for those who want to look great holding up an ice cold brew at Seamus' Ale House on Beer Belly Beach. You can't beat a workout that simultaneously produces both great physical appearance *and* peak field performance.

Like many of our other programs, this "look great—get it done" workout is user-friendly and versatile. It can easily be modified to enable you to work primarily on the development of either muscular strength and muscle size or muscular endurance. It's also designed to provide a significant and focused training stimulus for seasoned and less experienced lifters alike. If you want to focus primarily on developing muscular strength, size and power, then you should work through your sets using heavier weights and fewer repetitions; 3–5 repetitions per exercise would effectively promote this type of development. To the other end, firefighters who wish to enhance their abilities to extinguish multiple rooms of fire would be better off working on the development of muscular endurance. This can be accomplished by completing 15–20 repetitions with each exercise. Finally, a very popular approach in resistance training is to simultaneously work at improving muscular endurance, strength and size by completing 8–12 exercise repetitions. New lifters are encouraged to complete just one set and to move through the routine at a conservative pace. Experienced lifters should be able to handle multiple sets and proceed at a more deliberate pace.

1. Dumbbell One-Arm Row

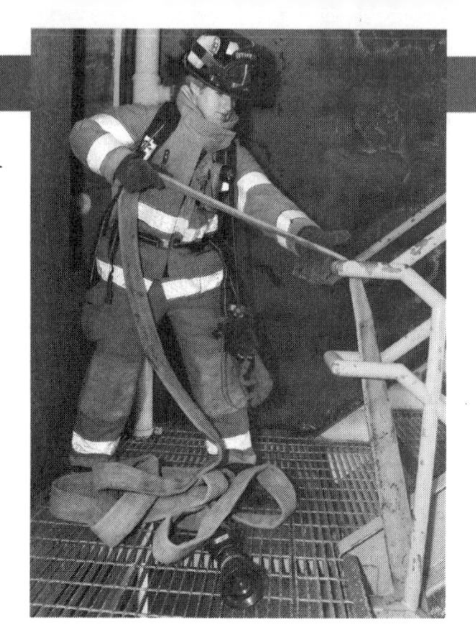

Imagine that you're pulling the hose line up the interior stairwell of a five-story building.

Target: Latissimus dorsi, teres major, posterior deltoid, rhomboids, trapezuis, biceps

Starting Position: Bend over and place one hand on a chair. Hold the weight with the other hand and let it hang to the ground. Keep your knees bent and your back straight.

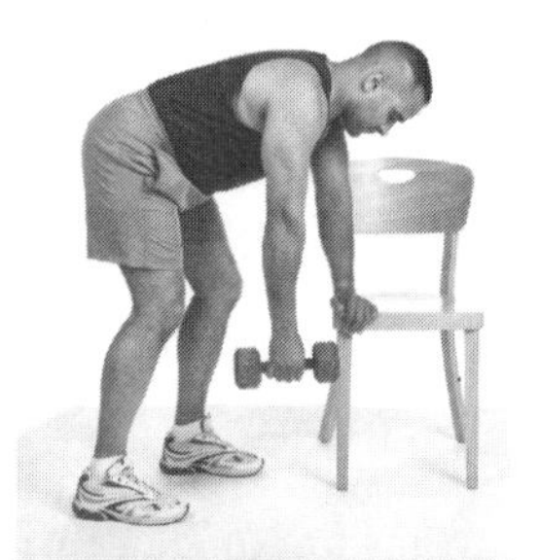

Starting Position

1 Leading with your elbow, lift the weight straight up and hold.

2 Slowly return to starting position.

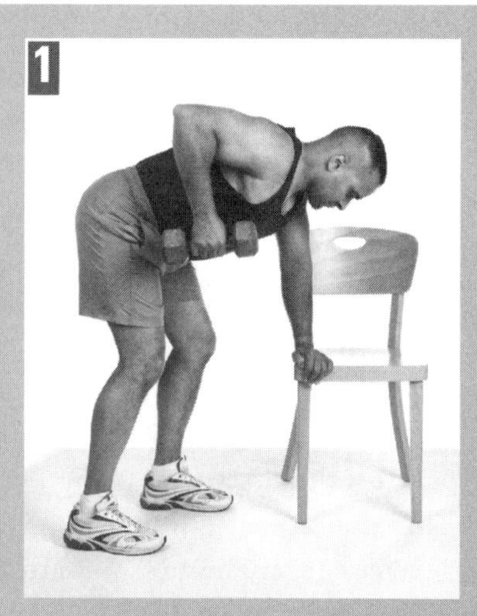

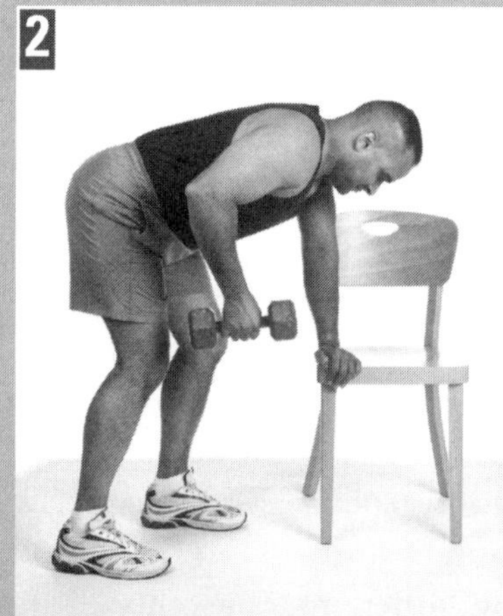

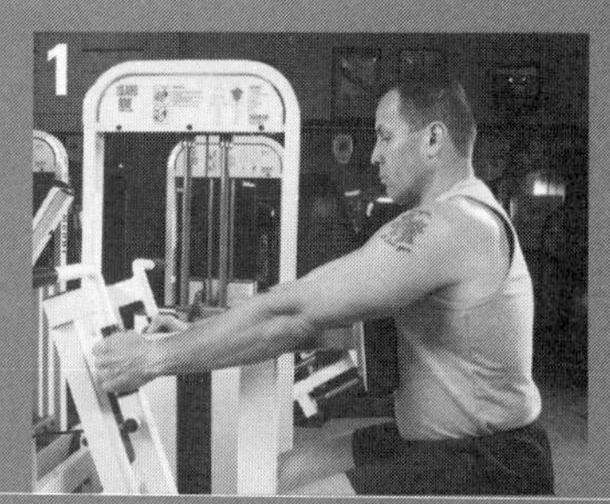

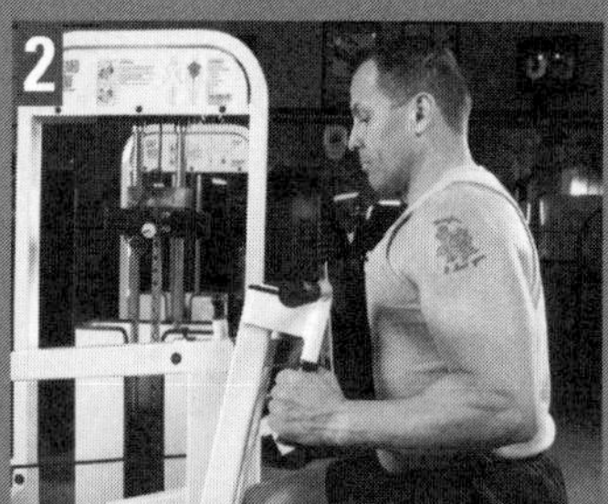

Alternative: Machine Compound Row

1 Sit facing the machine. Set the seat height so that the chest pad is at mid-chest level and your hands can just grab the vertical handles.

2 Pull the handles backward as far as possible and hold. Slowly return to starting position.

2. Combined Dumbbell Press

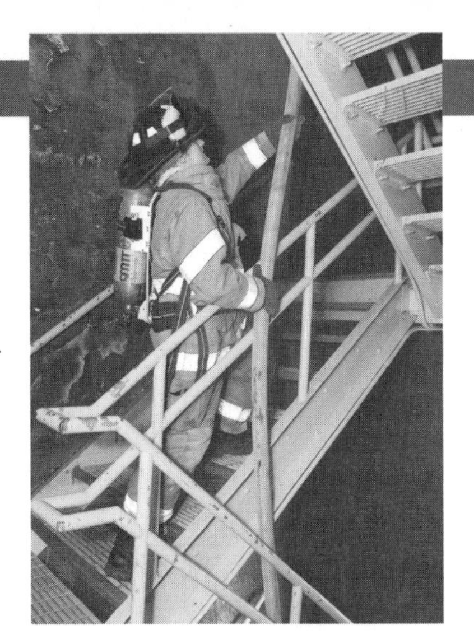

Imagine that you're feeding the hose line up the interior stairwell of a five-story building to allow advancement toward the fire.

Target: Deltoids, triceps

Starting Position: Stand with your feet staggered about shoulder-width apart. Stack the weights vertically (one on top of the other) at chest level.

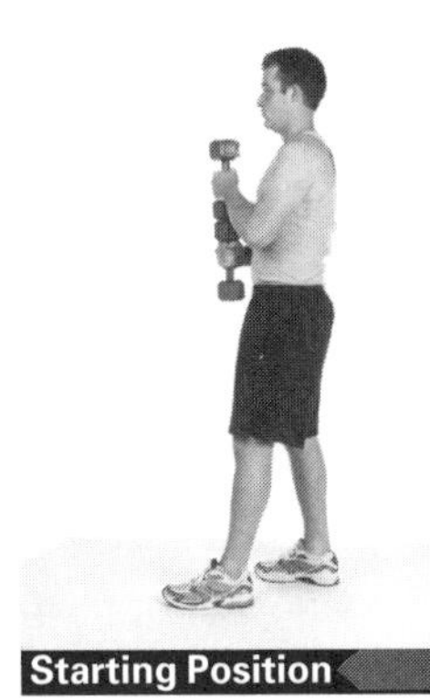

Starting Position

1. Press straight upward until your arms are almost fully extended and hold.
2. Slowly return to starting position.

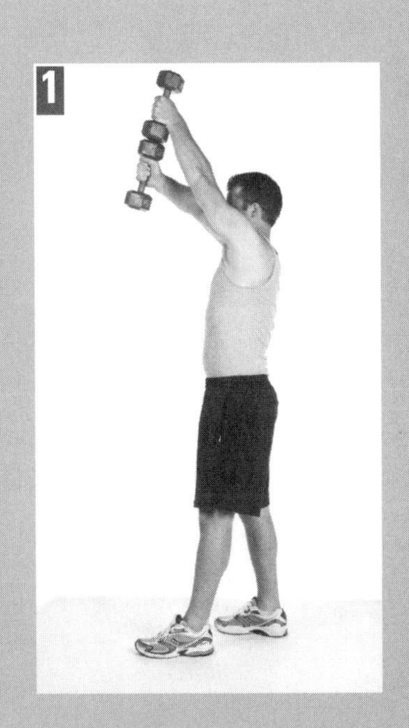

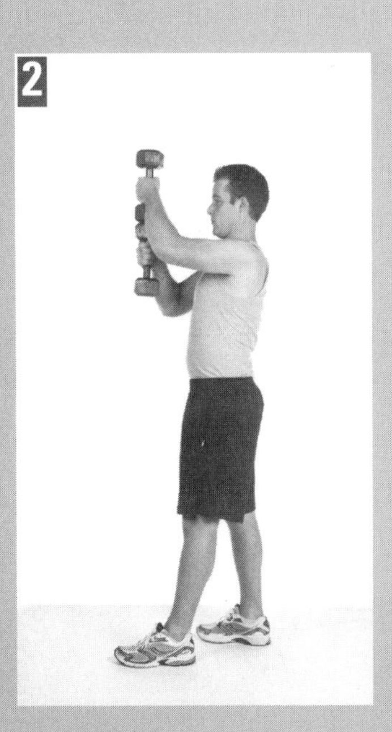

3. Dumbbell Curl

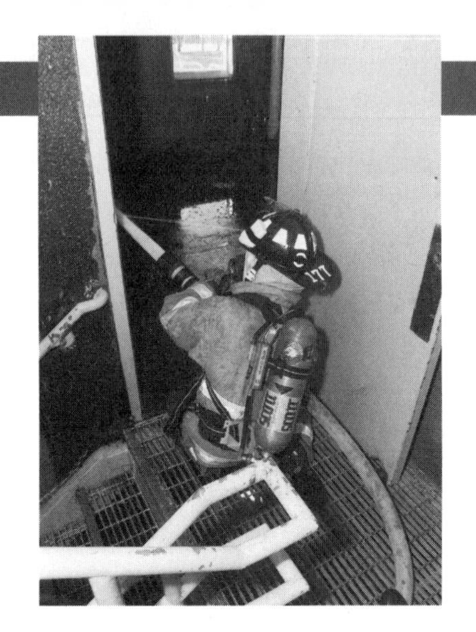

Imagine that you're approaching the apartment fire, feverishly rotating the nozzle of the hose in order to drive the fire back from the hallway.

Target: Biceps

Starting Position: Stand with your feet about shoulder-width apart, holding the weights at your sides with your palms facing forward.

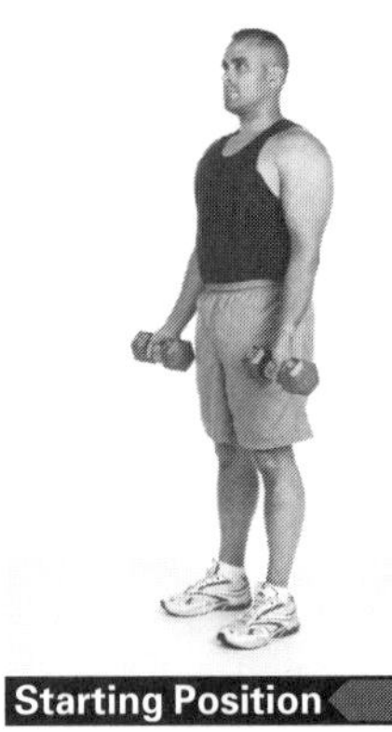

Starting Position

1. Bend your elbows to curl the weights toward your shoulders and hold.
2. Slowly return to starting position.

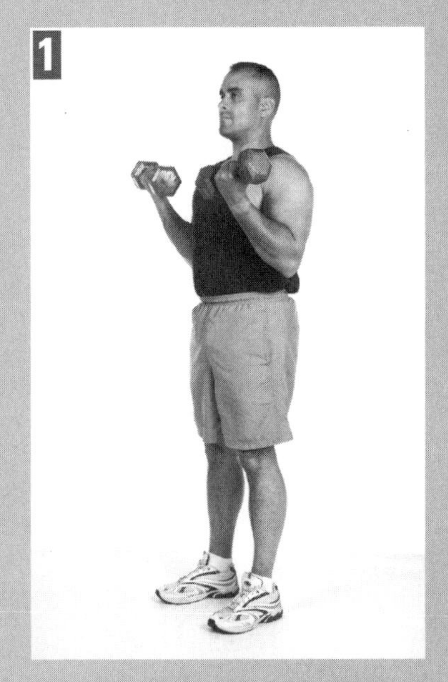

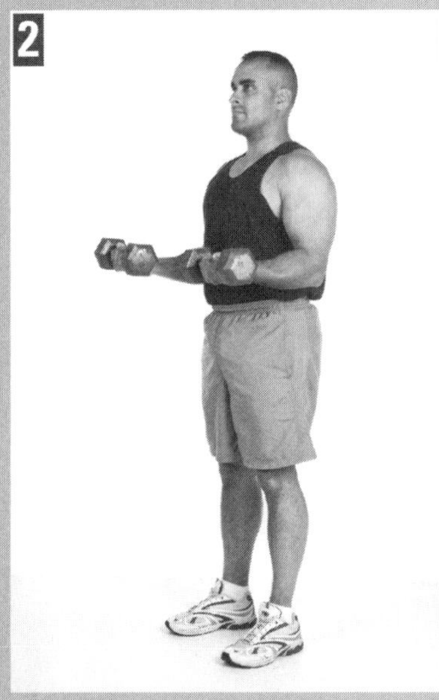

4. Dumbbell Kickback

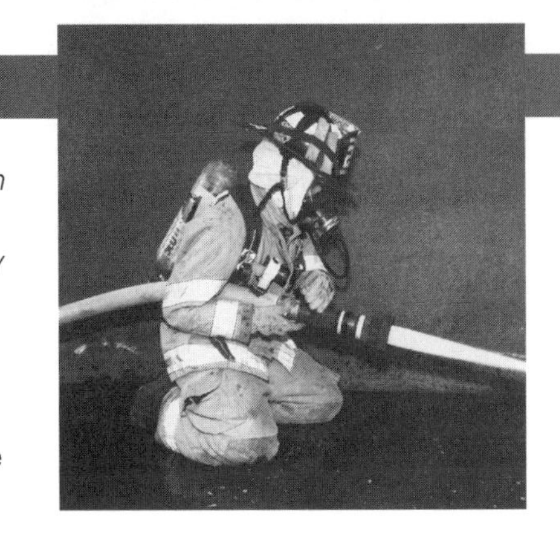

Imagine that you're operating the nozzle up toward the ceiling and then down toward the floor in order to cool the flooring surface, wash away any burning debris, and clear a path down the hallway to the main body of fire.

Target: Triceps

Starting Position: Bend over and place one hand on a chair. Hold the dumbbell in the other hand; your upper arm should be next to your side and your elbow should be bent at a 90-degree angle, with your lower arm directed downwards toward the ground.

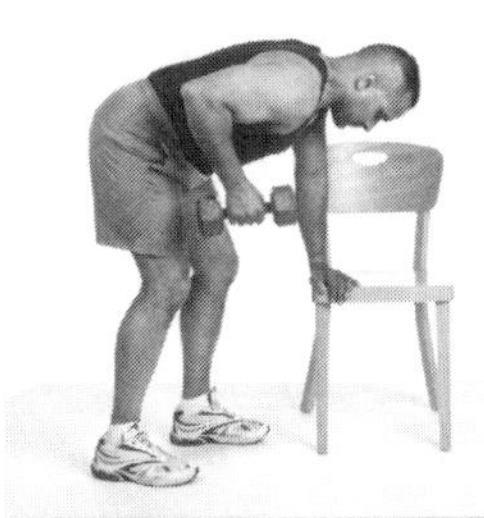

Starting Position

1. Keeping your upper arm next to your side, reach the weight back and straighten your elbow; hold.
2. Slowly return to starting position.

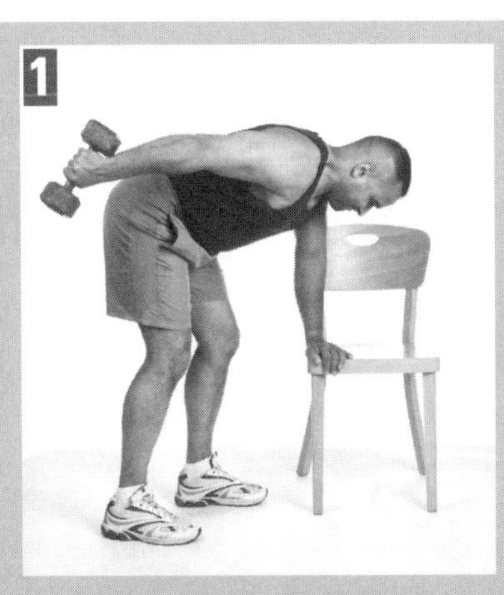

1

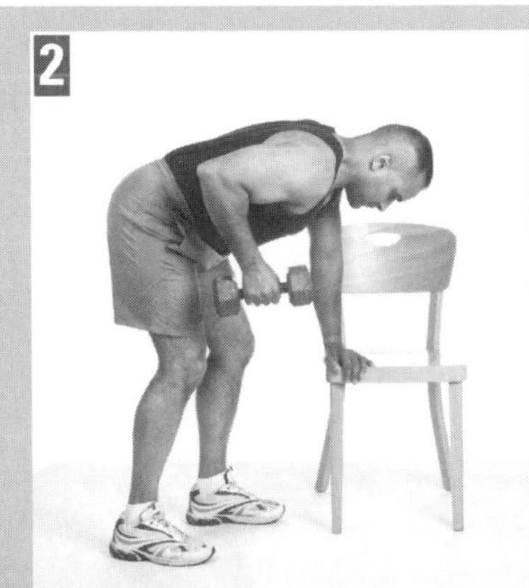

2

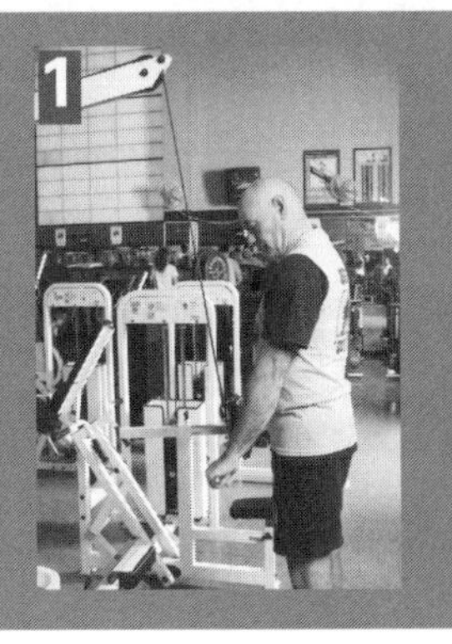

1

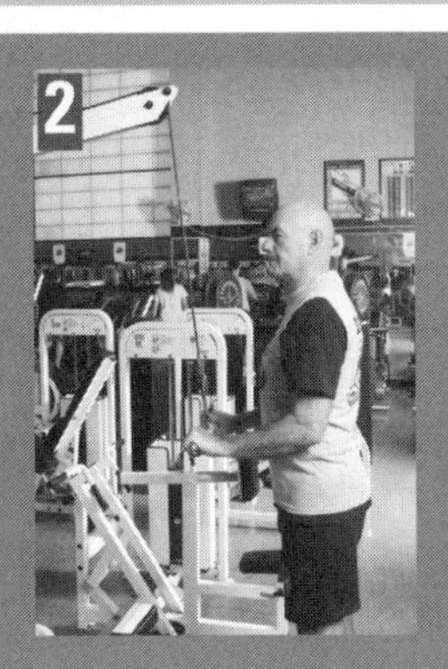

2

Alternative: Cable Triceps Press-Down

1. Stand with your feet about shoulder-width apart, facing the cable machine. Grasp the bar at chest level and keep your elbows at your sides.
2. Extend your arms downward until they are straight and hold. Slowly return to starting position.

5. Diagonal Incline Crunch

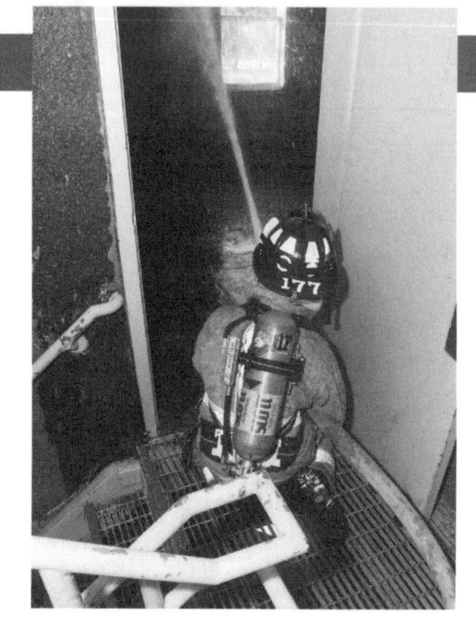

Imagine that you're extinguishing the fire left and right.

Target: Obliques, lower abdominals

Starting Position: Lie on an incline board with your hips bent and your feet hooked under the brace for support. Your shoulders should be in contact with the pad of the board.

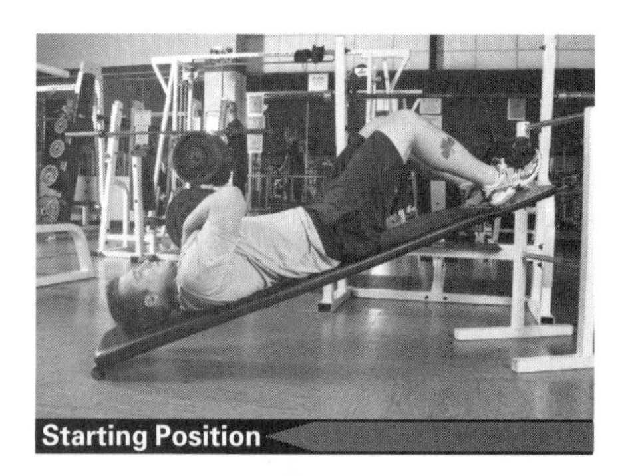
Starting Position

1. Curl your waist to raise your upper torso from the bench, moving your armpit to the opposite knee. Hold at the top.

2. Slowly return to starting position.

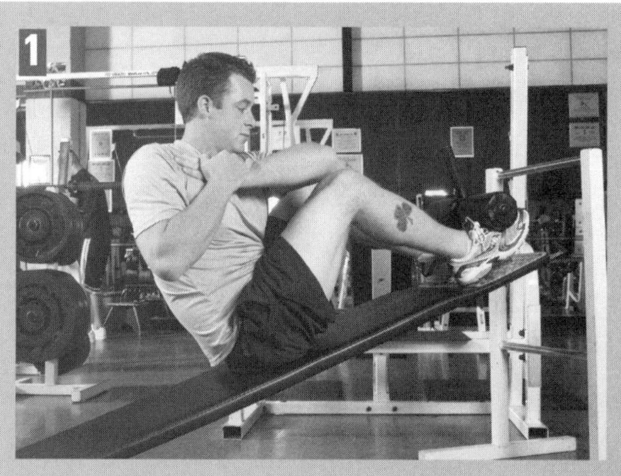
1

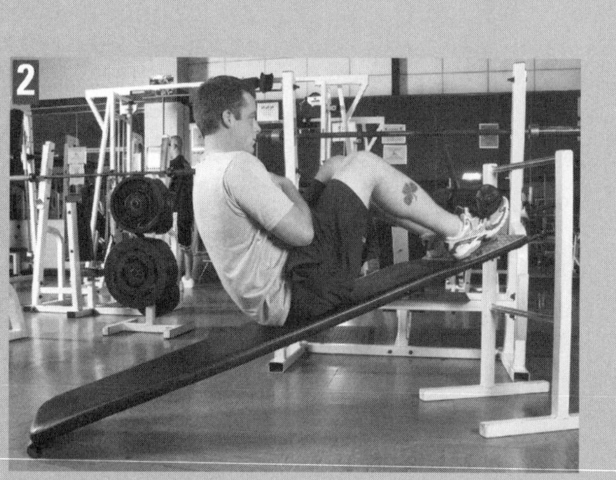
2

6. Dumbbell Fly

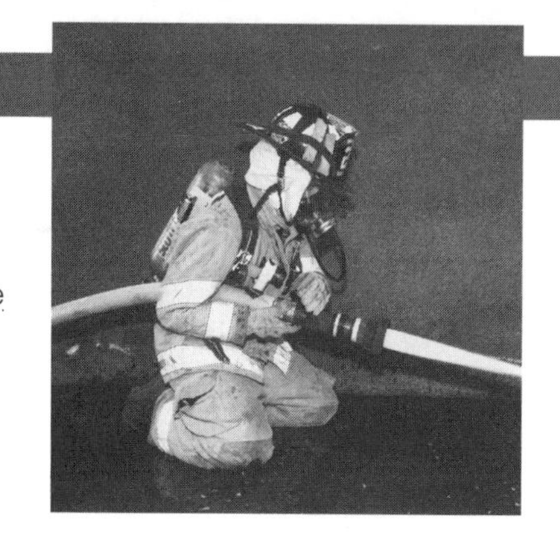

Imagine that you're extinguishing the fire along the floor.

Target: Pectorals

Starting Position: Lie on a bench, holding a weight in each hand. Raise them until they're directly above your chest; keep your elbows slightly bent.

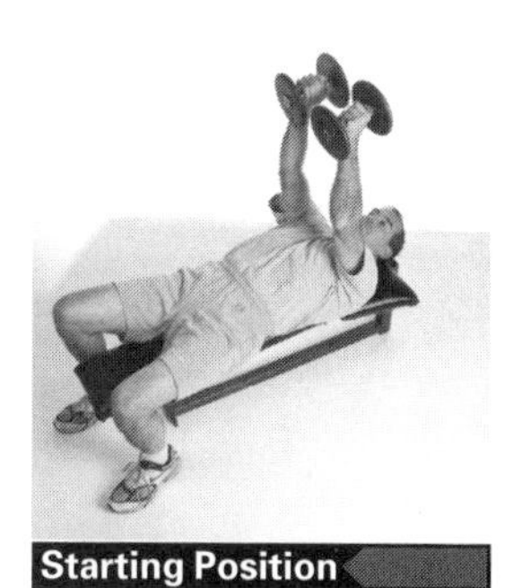

Starting Position

1. Slowly lower the weights in an arc straight out to the sides, maintaining a slight bend in your arms, and hold.
2. Slowly return to starting position.

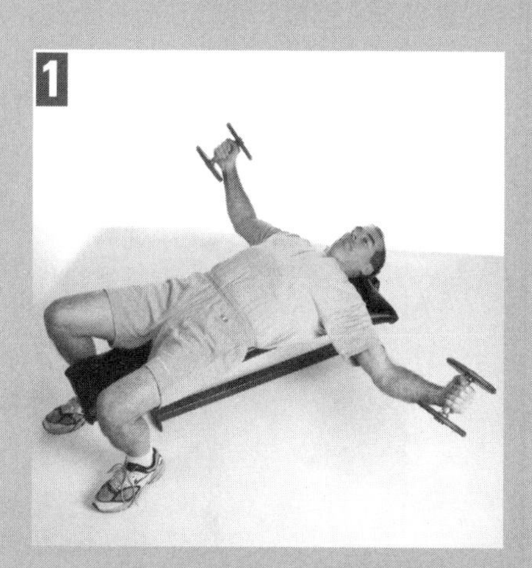

1

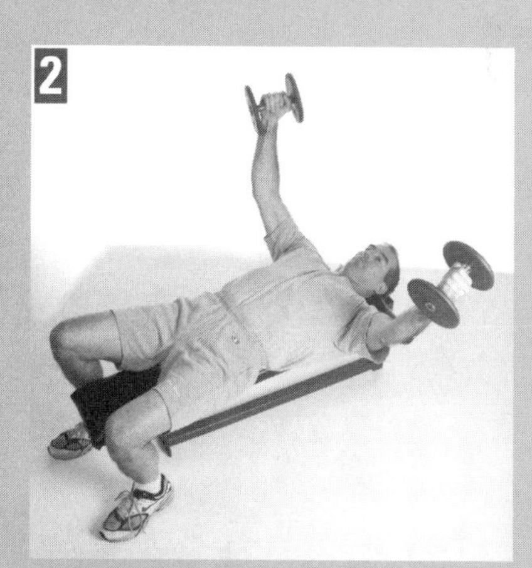

2

7. Back Extension

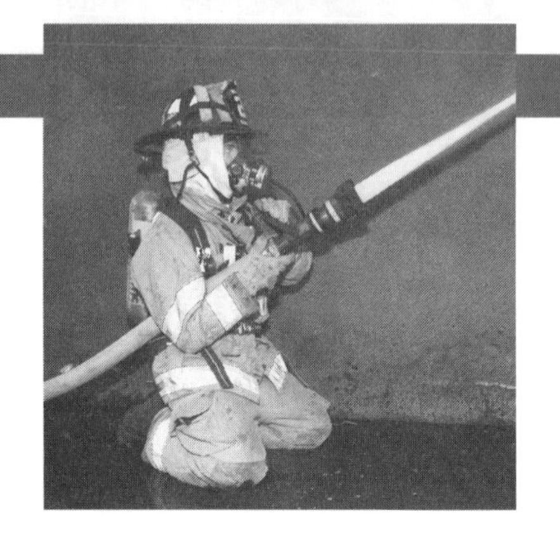

Imagine that you're extinguishing the fire on the ceiling and walls.

Target: Spinal erectors

Starting Position: Lie face down on the ground. Stack your hands on the floor and rest your chin on them.

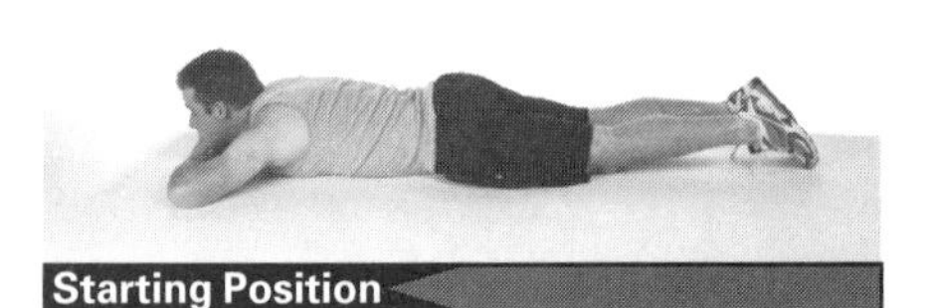
Starting Position

1. Slowly raise your arms and legs off the ground a few inches and hold.
2. Slowly return to starting position.

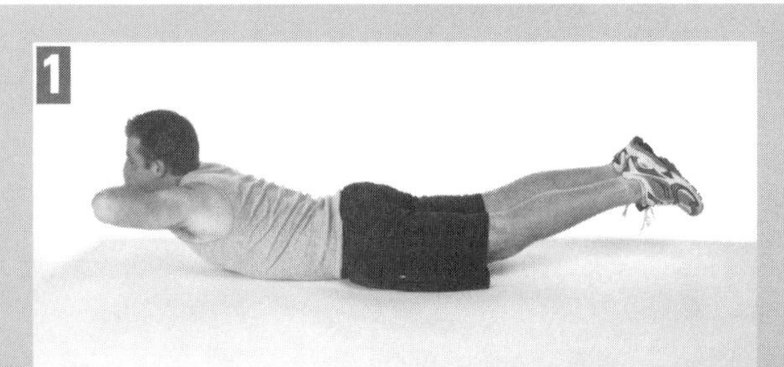

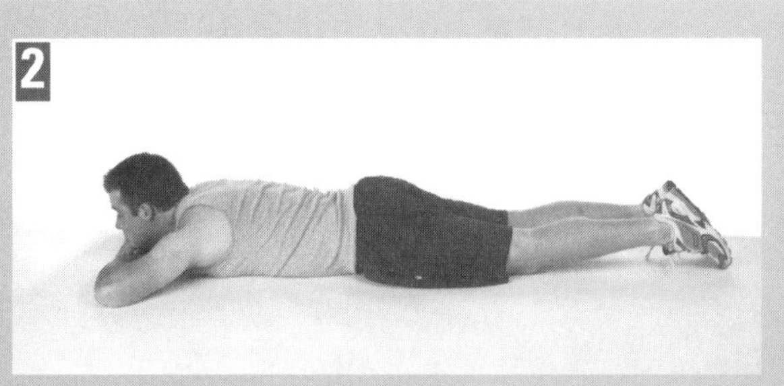

Alternative: Roman Chair—Back Extension

1. Lie face down and place your thighs on the large pad and your ankles under the support pads.
2. Bend at the waist and lower your body toward the floor. Raise and extend your waist and slowly return to starting position.

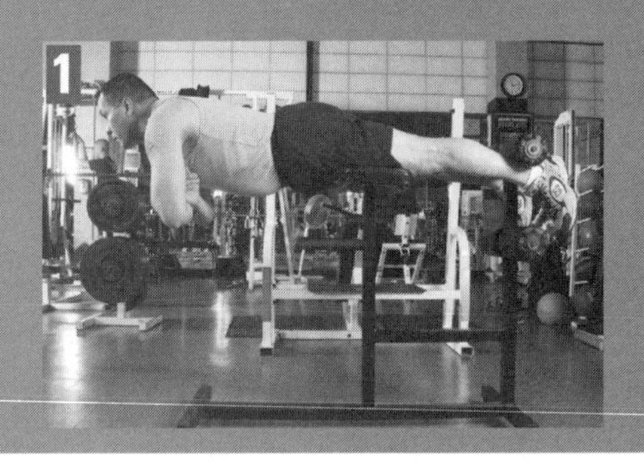

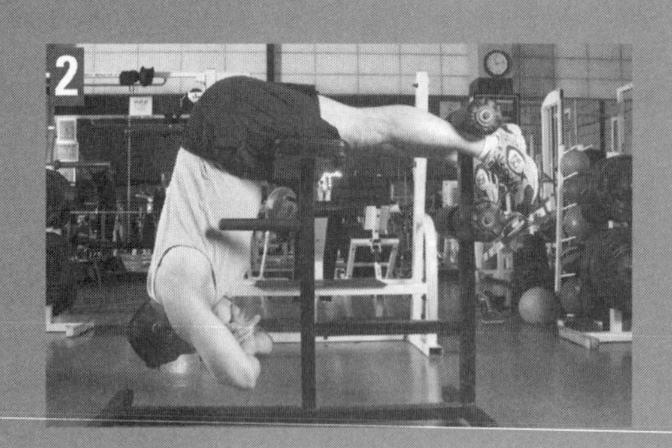

8. Dumbbell Reverse Curl

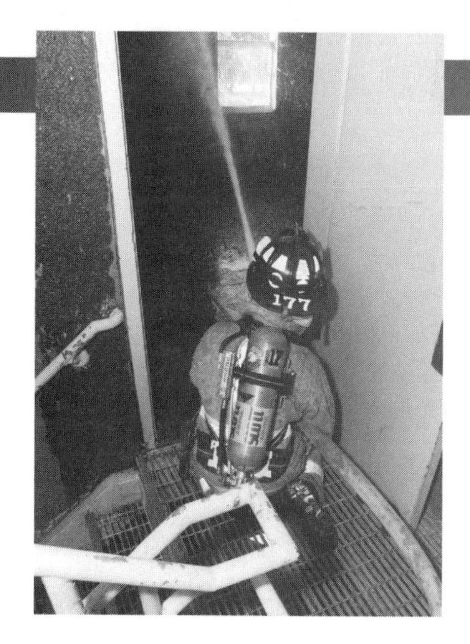

Imagine that you're knocking out those last few rooms of fire.

Target: Brachialis

Starting Position: Stand with your feet about shoulder-width apart, holding the weights with your palms facing your body.

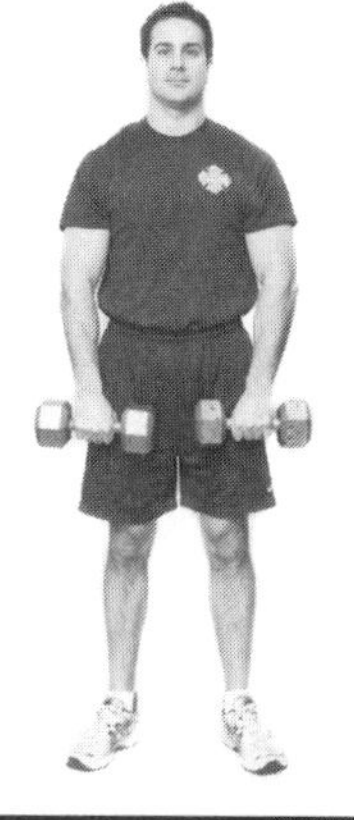

Starting Position

1. Bend your elbows to curl the weights toward your shoulders and hold.
2. Slowly return to starting position.

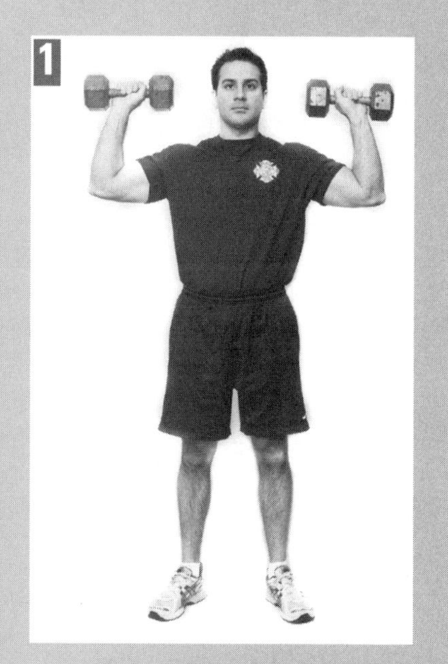

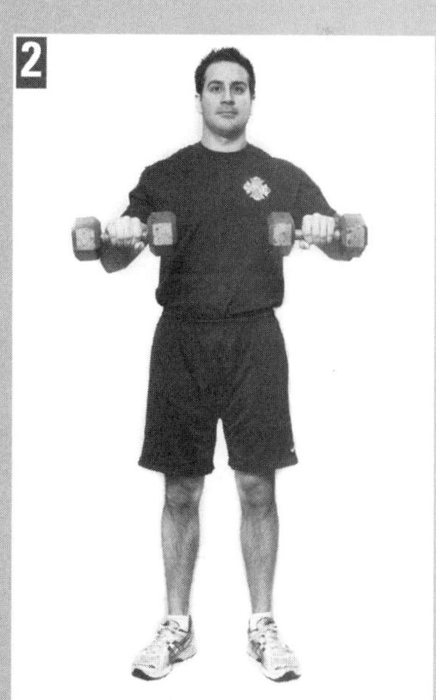

9. Dynaband Swing

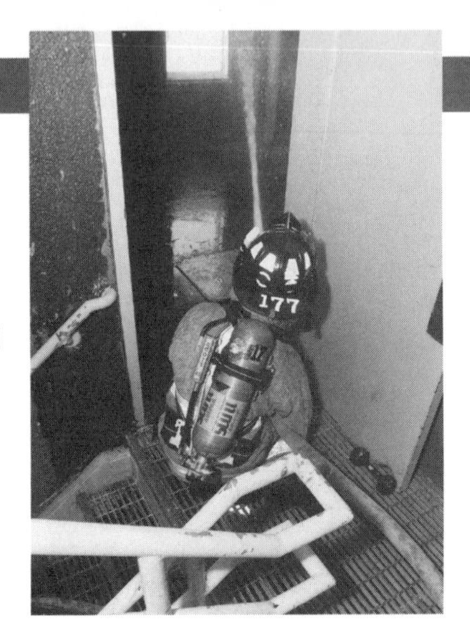

Imagine that you're hitting the fire left and right.

Target: Obliques, transverse abdominis

Starting Position: Tie the resistance band to an immovable object at a height between waist and chest level. Stand with your feet about shoulder-width apart and the resistance band to the side. Grasp the band with both hands. Take one step away to make sure the band is taut.

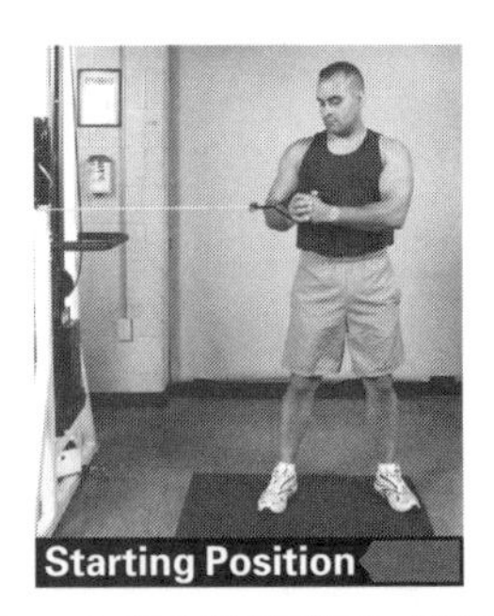
Starting Position

1. Turn your hips and trunk away from the immovable object.
2. Slowly return to starting position.

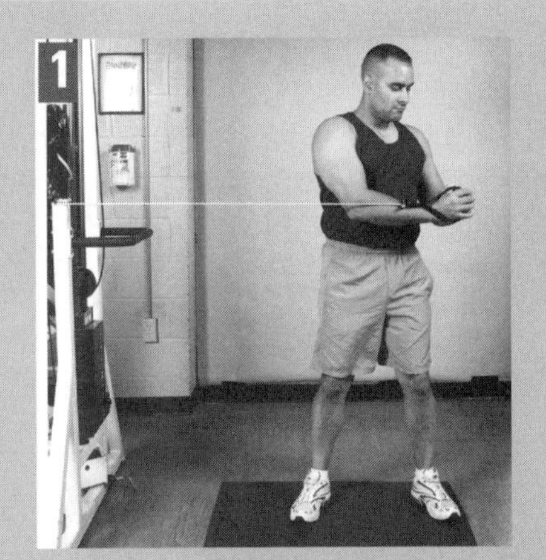

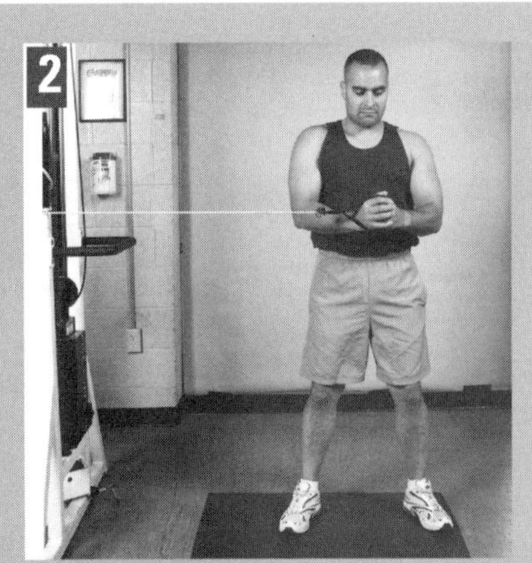

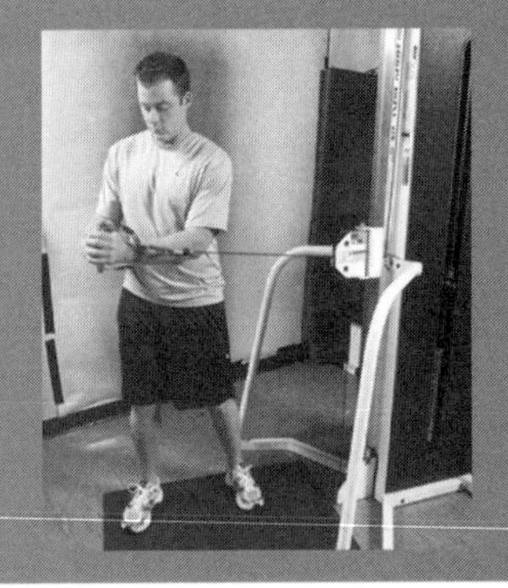

Alternative: Cable Swing

10. Dumbbell Wrist Roll

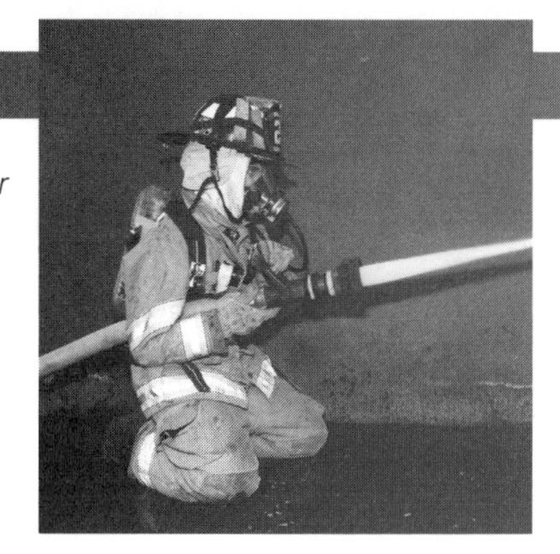

Imagine that you're squeezing the nozzle, directing the stream of water in all directions to extinguish the rest of the fire.

Target: Brachioradialis

Starting Position: Sitting on the edge of a chair or bench, grasp a weight in each hand and place your forearms and elbows on your thighs; your palms should face you. Lean forward.

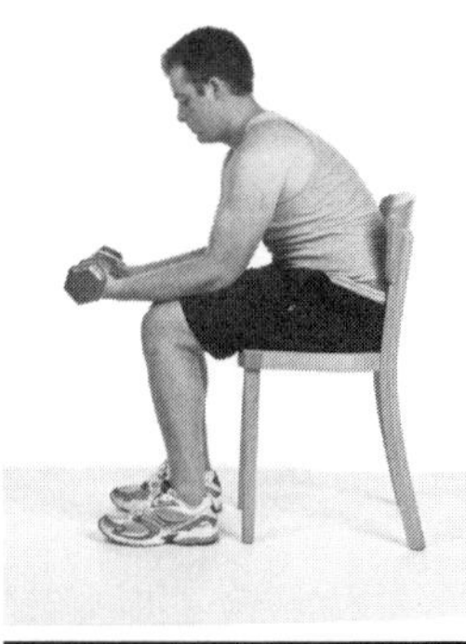

Starting Position

1 Flex your wrists toward the floor.

2 Return to starting position.

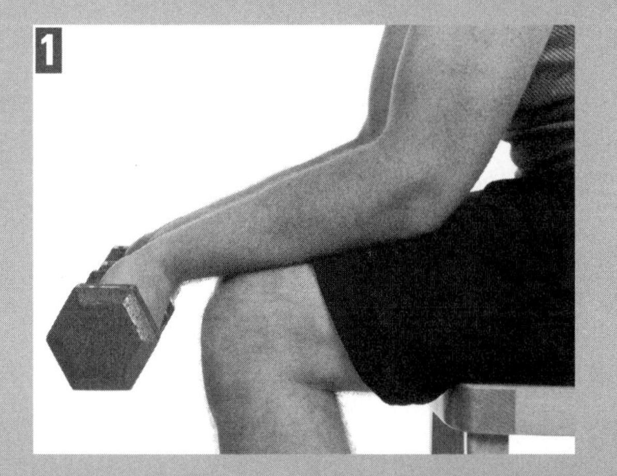

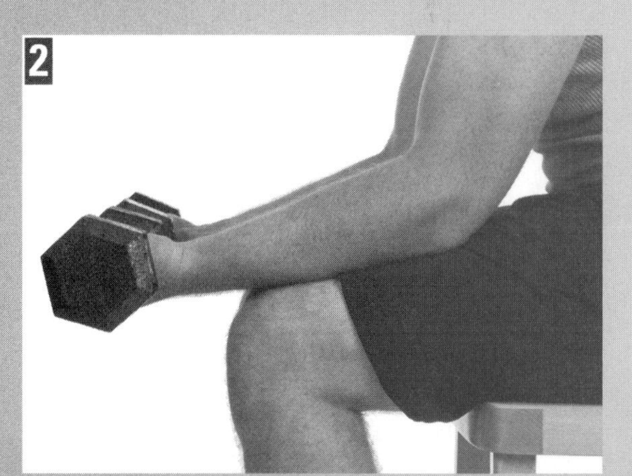

LADDER COMPANY CANMAN'S WORKOUT

The canman is a critical member of the interior search and rescue team. Carrying a six-foot pike pole and a two-and-a-half-gallon water extinguisher ("can"), the canman forces open doors, extinguishes fire, rescues victims, and opens holes in the ceiling and walls to inspect for extending fire. This firefighter's primary responsibility is to save lives, so the need for peak muscular fitness is clear and apparent. The canman position is often assigned to the newest member of a ladder company, so if you're aspiring to become a firefighter or have just recently been appointed, this is the ideal workout for you. It's also an excellent workout for athletes involved in physical activities that rely heavily on powerful upper body strength, and fitness-oriented individuals who enjoy the look and feel of a powerhouse firefighter/athlete.

The program focuses on arm, shoulder and body core development. The triceps are emphasized, so profile-quality horseshoes (triceps) and dynamic arm-pushing power are bound to result. Remember, if you're looking to increase muscle size in the arms, shoulders and chest, you should use heavier weights and complete fewer repetitions. If you're a firefighter looking to develop muscular endurance, then more repetitions and the use of moderate weight is the way to go. Unless you're an experienced lifter, we recommend that you complete just one exercise set in the first few training sessions. It would also be a good idea to start out using light weights, to complete either 8–12 or 15–20 repetitions with each exercise and to take adequate time for near-complete recovery between exercises (1–2 minutes). Grant your body some time to get used to this new and intense type of physical challenge. Then build as your strength and/or muscular endurance improve. Experienced lifters should complete either 2 or 3 sets.

This program is going to take your triceps to the limit and get you in the kind of shape it takes to operate at peak levels in the fire field as a high-performance ladder company canman.

1. Dumbbell Curl & Press

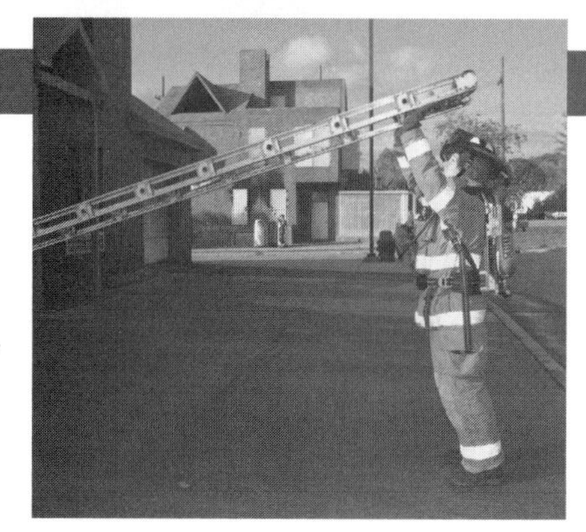

Imagine that you're lifting the tip of the ladder up and pressing it over your head.

Target: Anterior deltoid, brachialis, triceps

Starting Position: Stand with your feet about shoulder-width apart, holding the weights at your sides, palms facing inward.

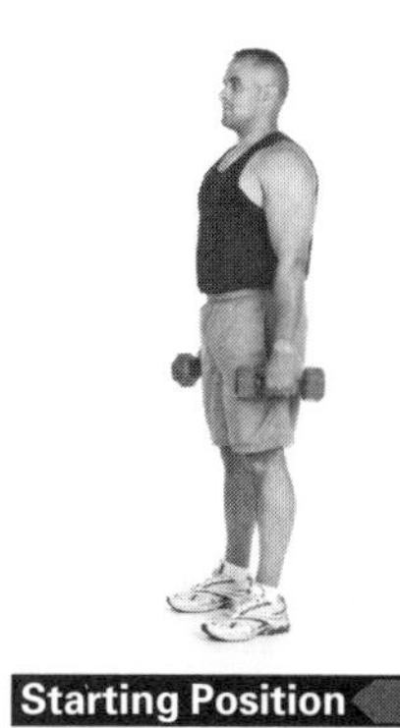

Starting Position

1. Bend your elbows to curl the weights to your shoulders.
2. Then press the weights overhead until your arms are almost fully extended.
3. Slowly return to starting position.

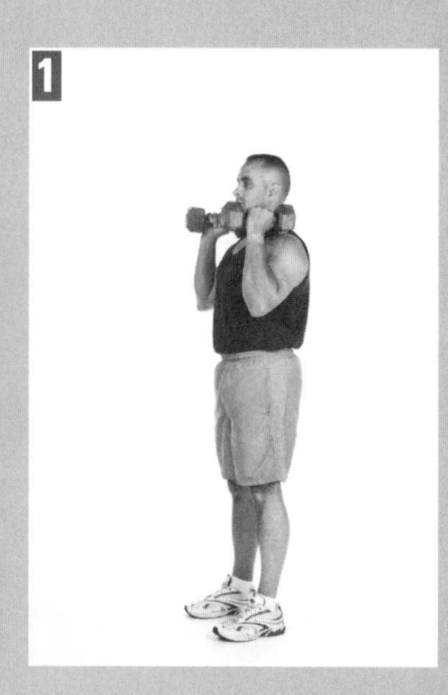

1

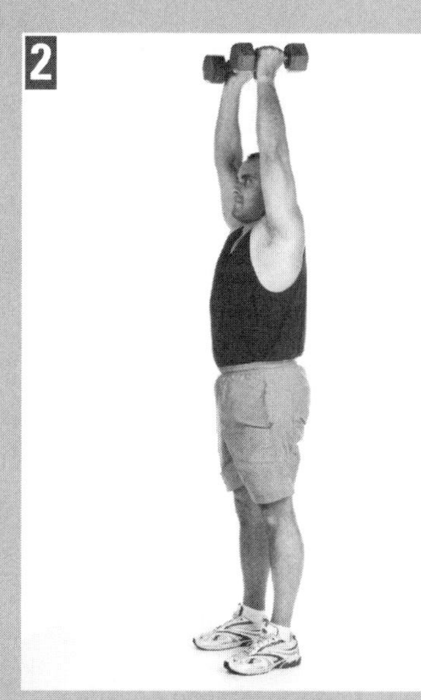

2

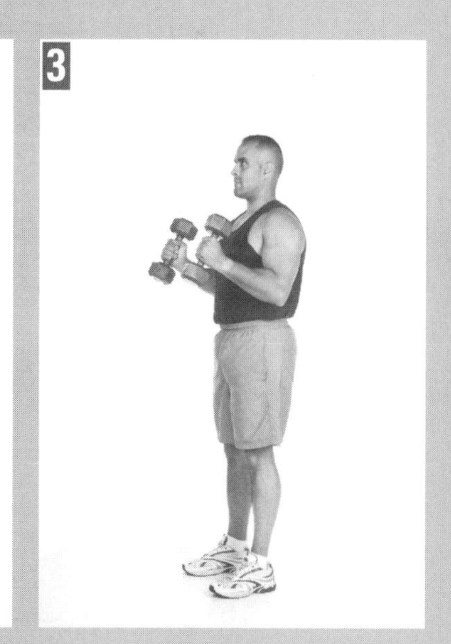

3

2. Cable Rope Pull-Down

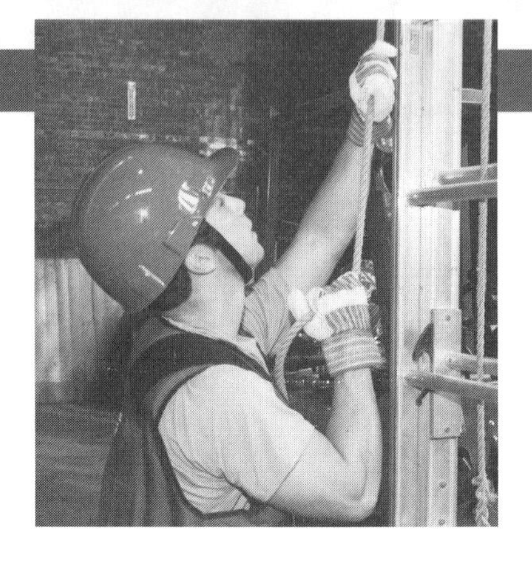

Imagine that you're pulling on the ladder rope (halyard) to extend the fly section of the portable ladder up to the second floor of an apartment building.

Target: Latissimus dorsi, biceps

Starting Position: Stand with your feet about shoulder-width apart. Grasp the rope with one hand above the other, making sure your arms are almost fully extended.

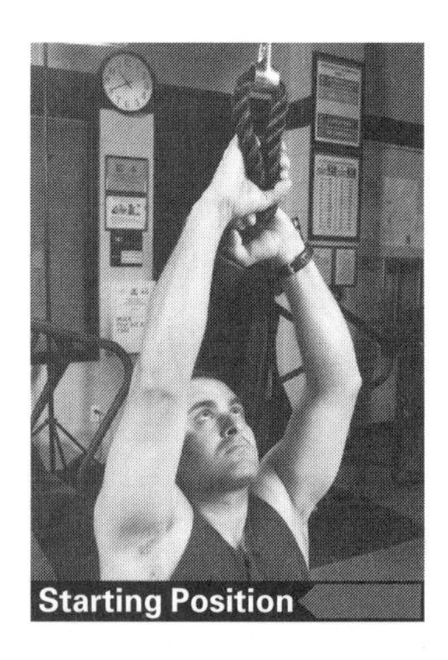
Starting Position

1. Pull downward on the rope, using your upper hand to do most of the work. Hold.

2. Slowly return to starting position and then repeat the exercise, emphasizing the use of your other hand.

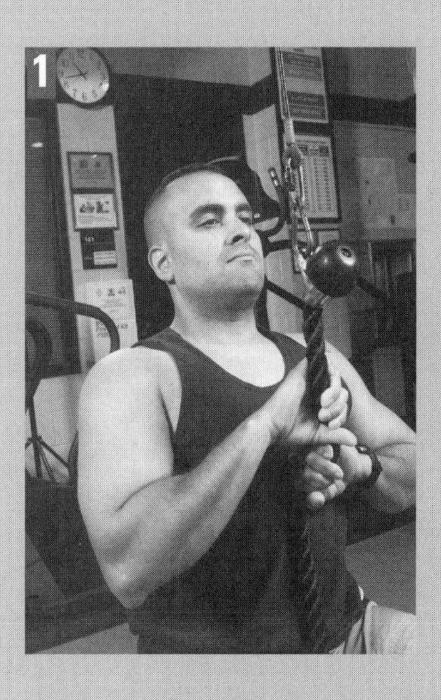
1

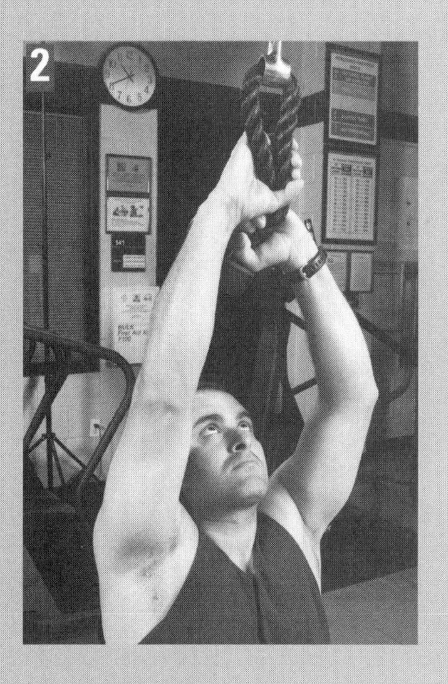
2

3. Dynaband Swing

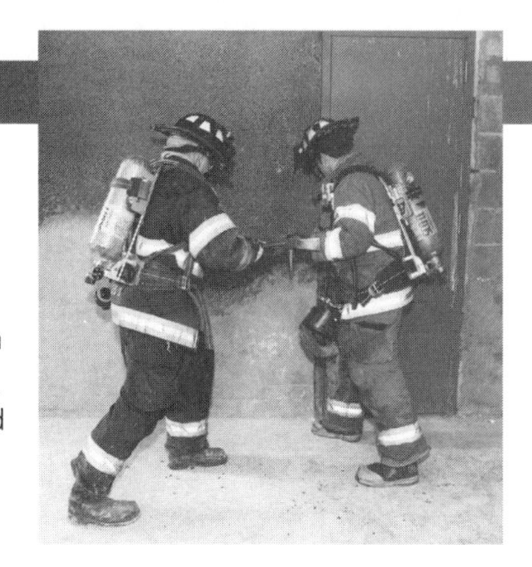

Imagine that you're swinging the maul to drive the fork end of the Halligan through the seam of the apartment door.

Target: Obliques, tranverse abdominis

Starting Position: Tie the resistance band to an immovable object at a height between waist and chest level. Stand with your feet about shoulder-width apart and the resistance band to the side. Grasp the band with both hands. Take one step away to make sure the band is taut.

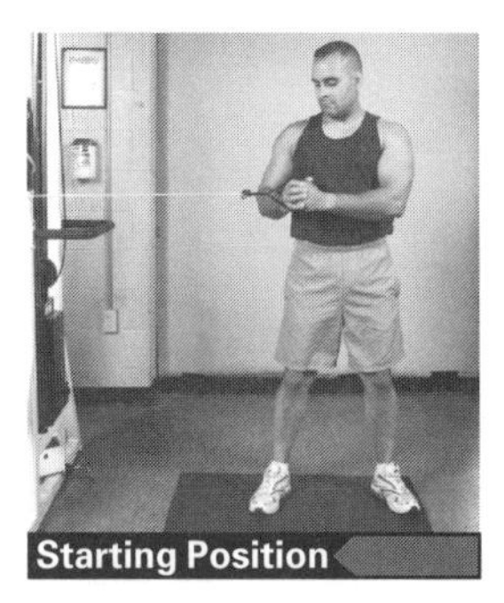
Starting Position

1. Turn your hips and trunk away from the immovable object. Hold.
2. Slowly return to starting position.

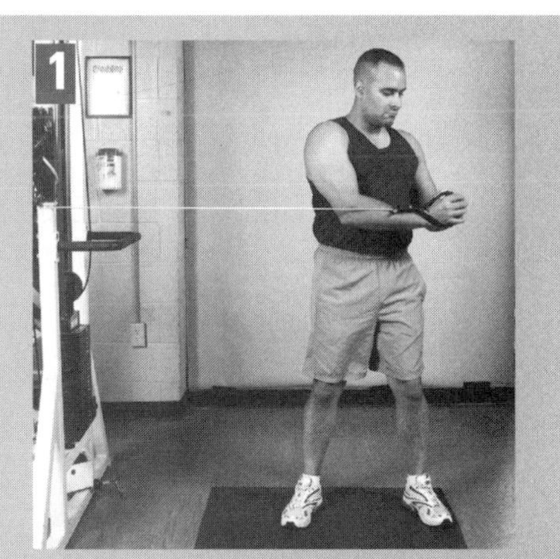
1

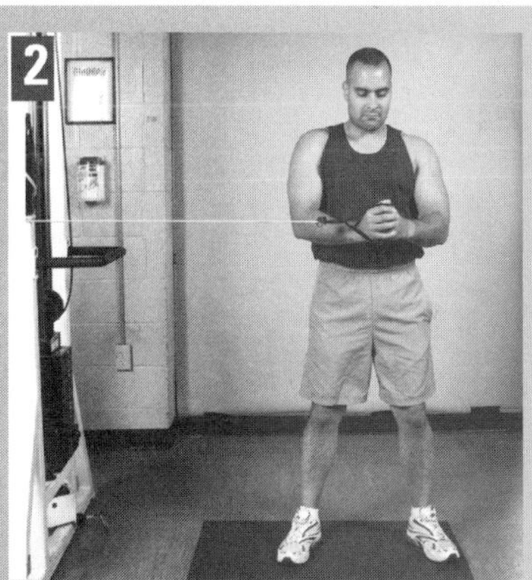
2

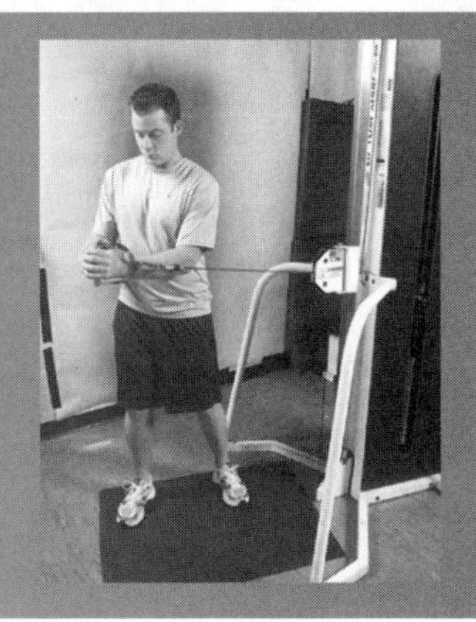

Alternative: Cable Swing

4. Dumbbell Bench Press

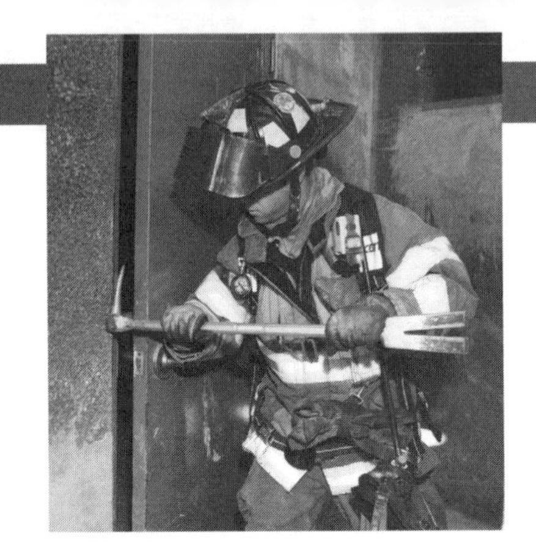

Imagine that you're pushing forcefully on the Halligan to force open a door that opens outwards.

Target: Pectorals

Starting Position: Sit on a bench with the weights resting on your lower thighs. Lie down. Position the dumbbells to the sides of your upper chest with your elbows directly under the weights.

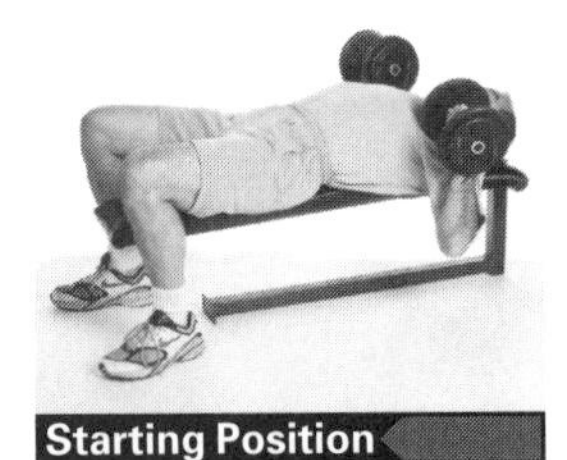
Starting Position

1. Press the weights straight up, keeping your elbows at your sides, until your arm are almost fully extended.
2. Slowly return to starting position.

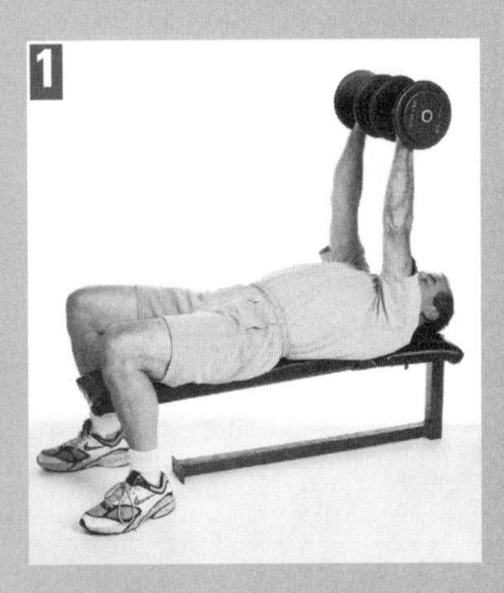
1

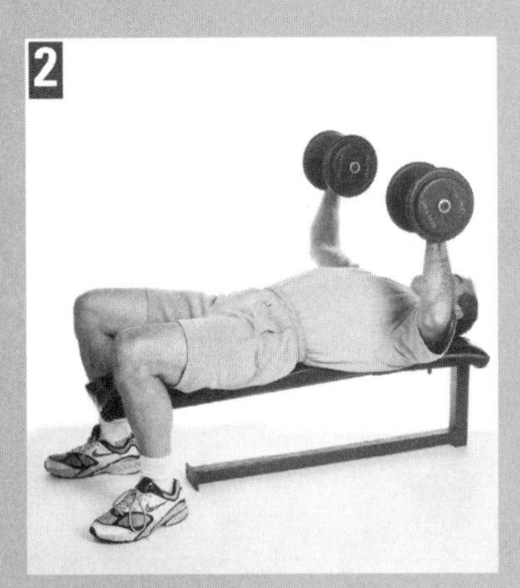
2

5. Dumbbell One-Arm Row

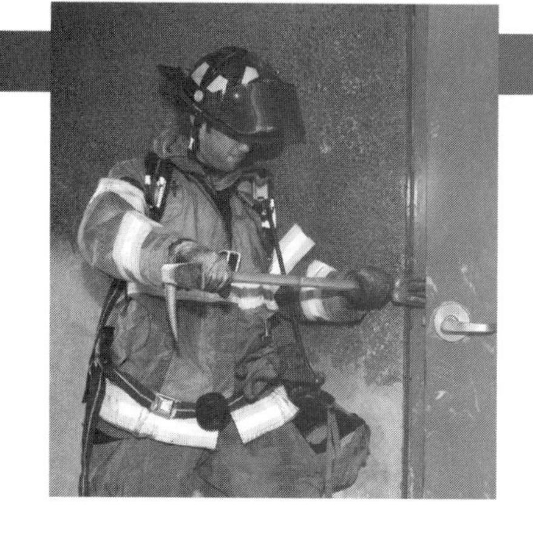

Imagine that you're pulling forcefully on the Halligan to force open a door that opens outward.

Target: Latissimus dorsi, teres major, posterior deltoid, rhomboids, trapezuis, biceps

Starting Position: Bend over and place one hand on a chair. Hold the weight with the other hand and let it hang to the ground. Keep your knees bent and your back straight.

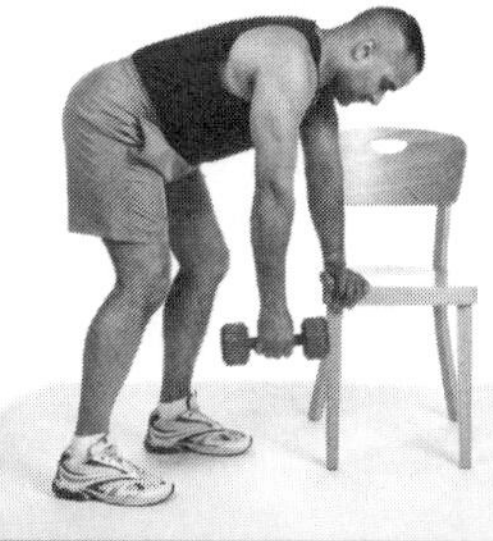

Starting Position

1 Leading with your elbow, lift the weight straight up and hold.

2 Slowly return to starting position.

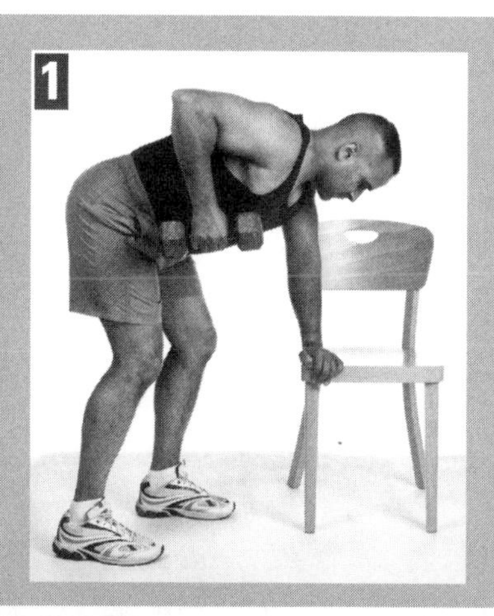

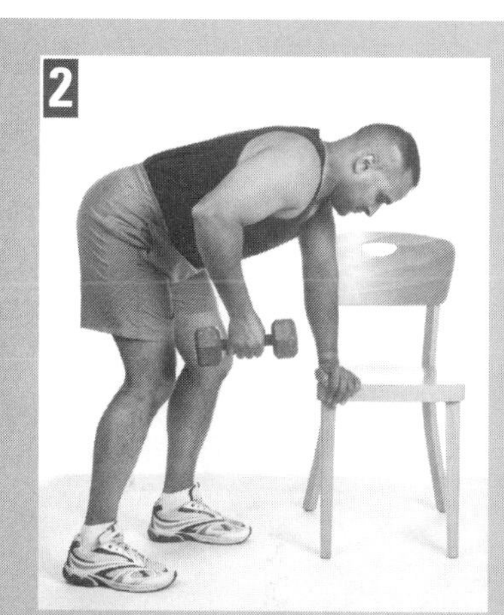

Alternative: Cable Low Row

1 Sit facing the machine so that your legs are extended but still slightly bent. Grab the handles, making sure your arms are completely straight.

2 Pull the handles backward as far as possible and hold. Slowly return to starting position.

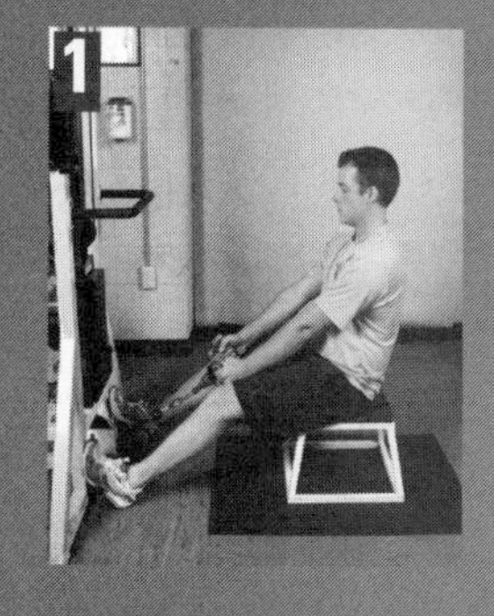

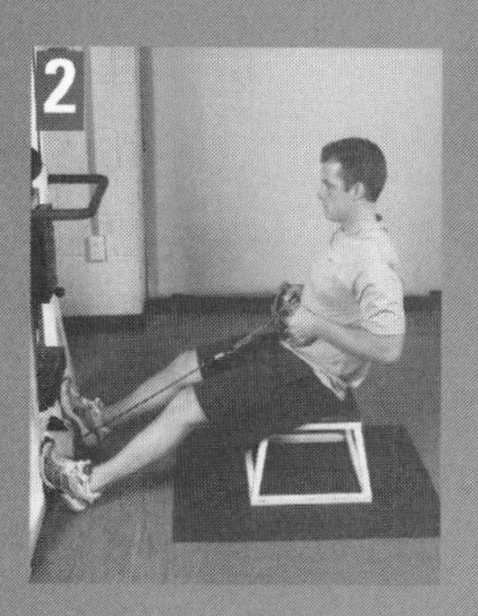

6. Crunch

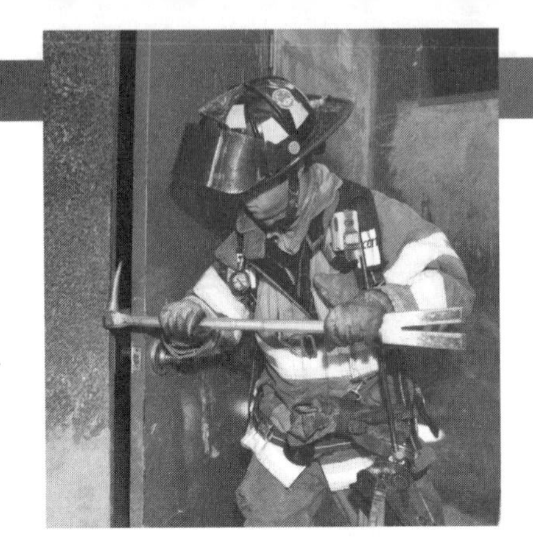

Imagine that you're forcibly working the door to get inside the apartment and search for trapped or unconscious victims.

Target: Rectus abdominis

Starting Position: Lie on your back and bend your knees to about 90 degrees, placing your feet flat on the floor. Fold your arms across your chest.

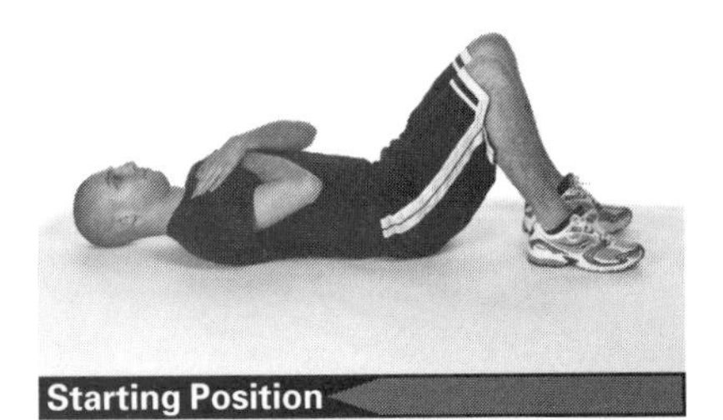
Starting Position

1 Slowly raise your shoulders a few inches off the ground and hold.

2 Slowly return to starting position.

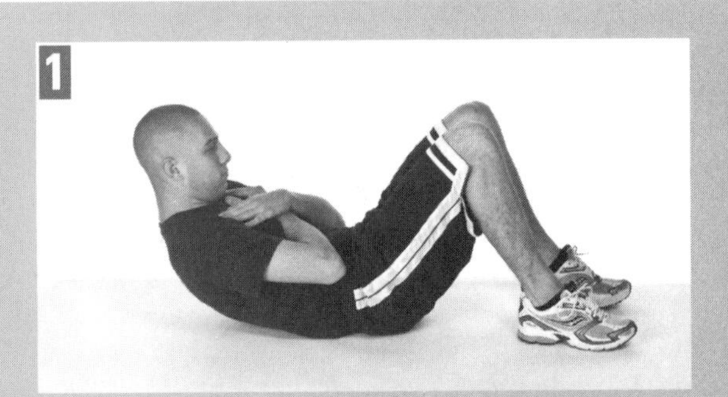
1

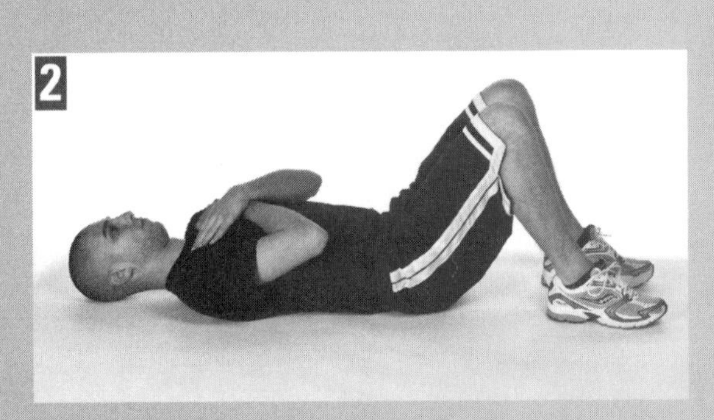
2

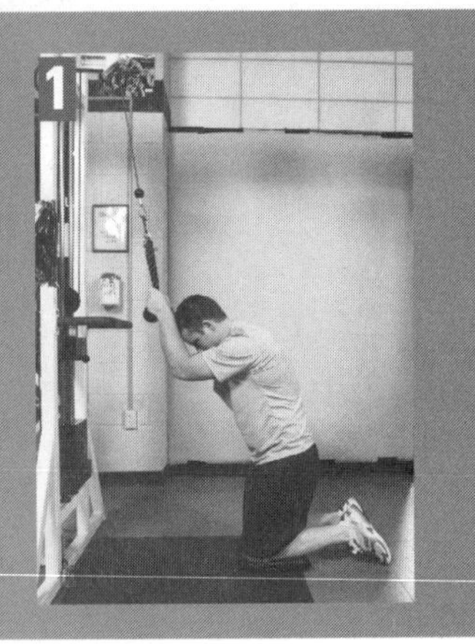
1

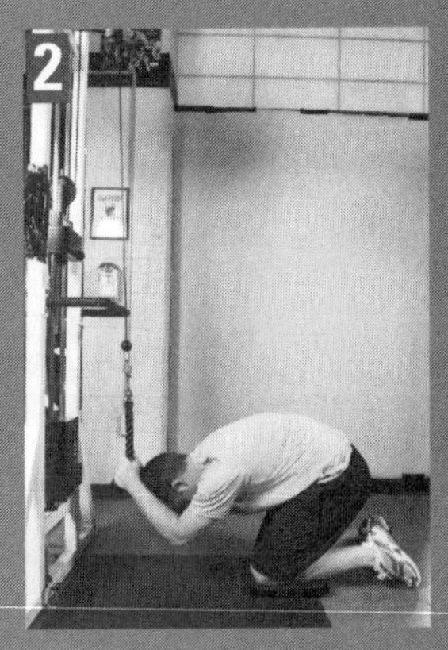
2

Alternative: Cable Crunch

1 Stand or kneel in front of a high pulley and grip a bar with an underhand grip or use a rope (as pictured). Hold the bar so your wrists are close to your ears. Arch your back slightly.

2 Crunch your elbows downward, pivoting at the bottom of your rib cage, not at the waist. Squeeze hard, then rise up until your back is arched again in the starting position.

7. Back Extension

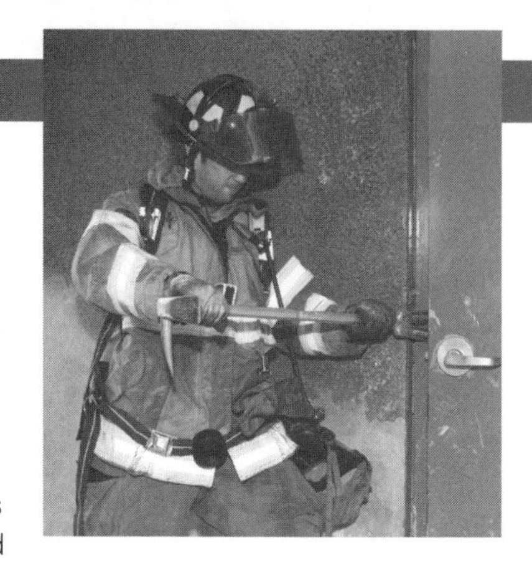

Imagine that you're executing powerful and dynamic forcible entry movements to get inside the apartment.

Target: Spinal erectors

Starting Position: Lie face down on the ground. Stack your hands on the floor and rest your chin on them.

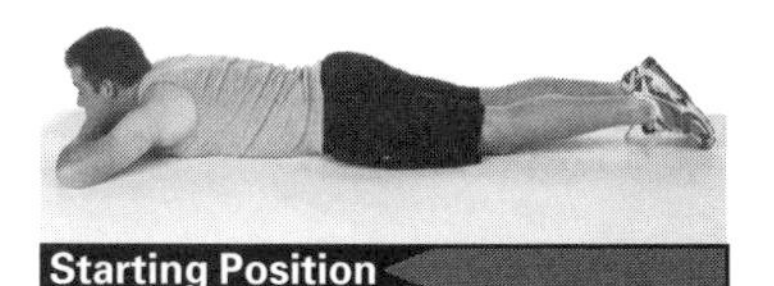

Starting Position

1. Slowly raise your arms and legs off the ground a few inches and hold.
2. Slowly return to starting position.

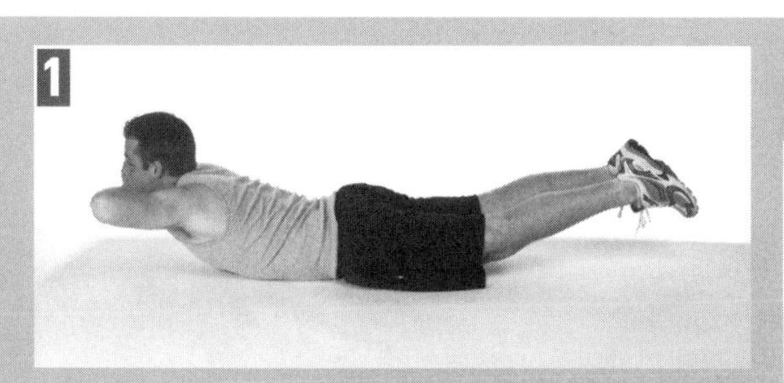

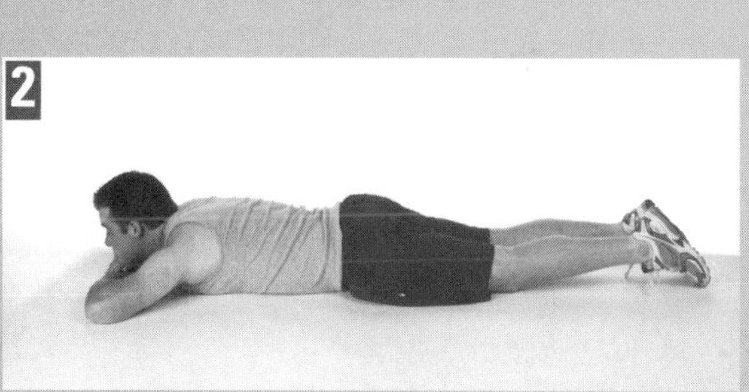

Alternative: Roman Chair—Back Extension

1. Lie face down and place your thighs on the large pad and your ankles under the support pads.
2. Bend at the waist and lower your body toward the floor. Raise and extend your waist and slowly return to starting position.

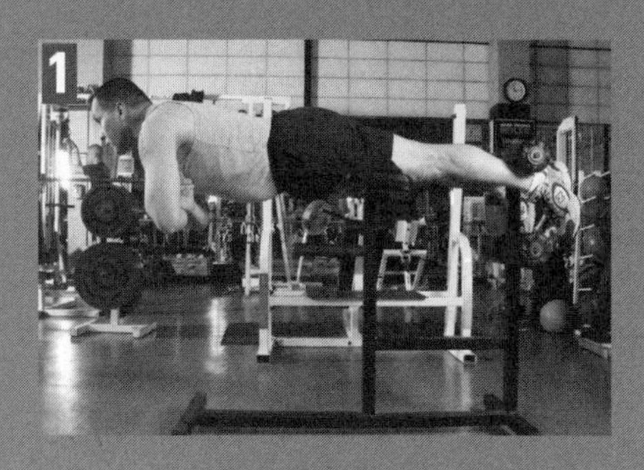

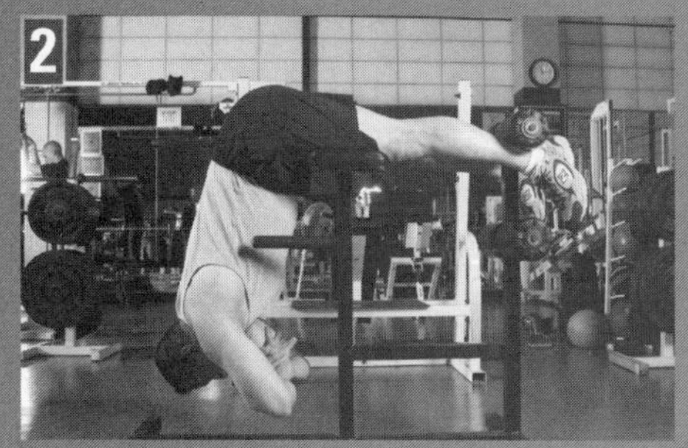

8. Combined Dumbbell Press

Imagine that you're driving the six-foot pike pole up into the ceiling to inspect for any extension of fire.

Target: Deltoids, triceps

Starting Position: Stand with your feet staggered about shoulder-width apart. Stack the weights vertically (one on top of the other) at chest level.

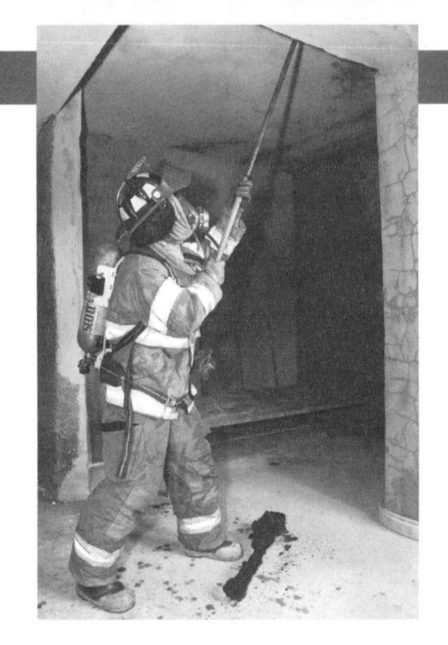

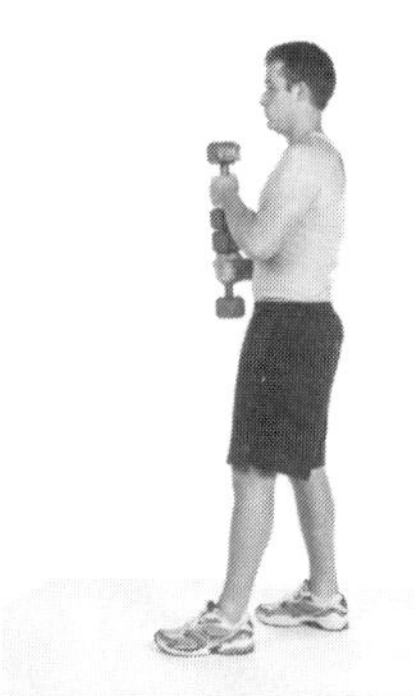

Starting Position

1. Press straight upward until your arms are almost fully extended and hold.
2. Slowly return to starting position.

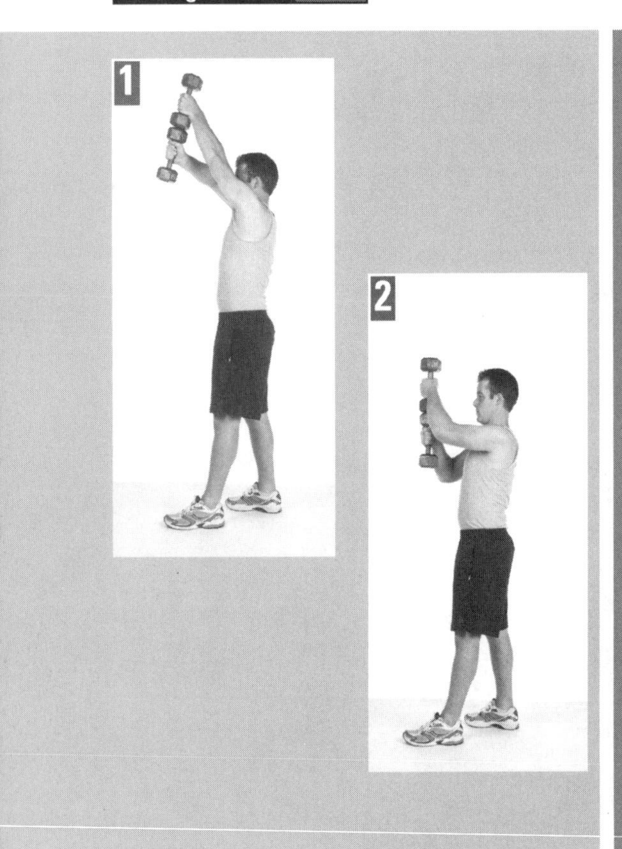

Alternative: Cable Lift & Press (Vertical Bar)

1. Stand facing the cable machine with the cable at the "low" position. Hold the straight curl bar in a vertical position with your arms slightly bent.
2. Press the bar up toward the ceiling. Slowly return to starting position.

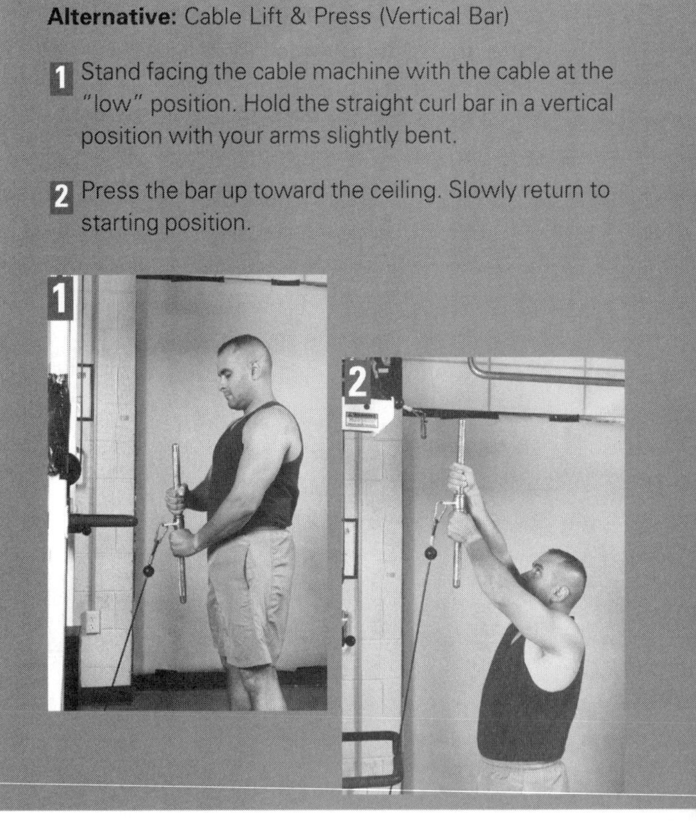

9. Cable Pull-Down (Vertical Bar)

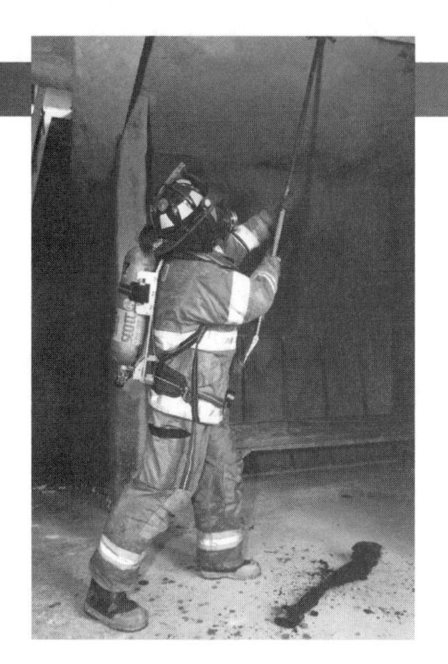

Imagine that you're grabbing hold of the ceiling boards and pulling them down to inspect the ceiling for any extension of fire.

Target: Latissimus dorsi, biceps

Starting Position: Stand facing the cable machine with the cable at the "high" position. Hold the straight curl bar in a vertical position with your arms slightly bent.

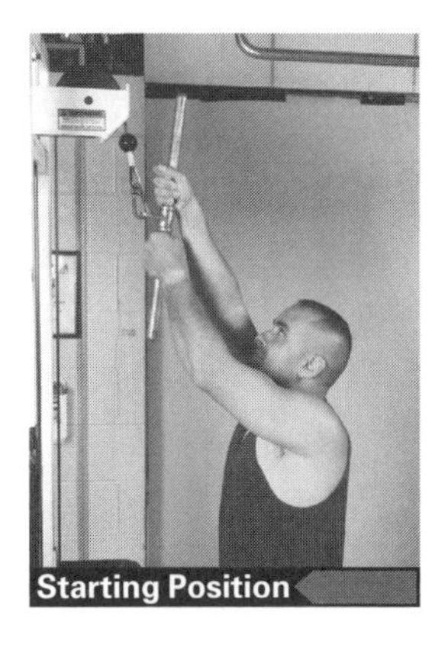

Starting Position

1. Pull the bar down toward your mid-section.
2. Slowly return to starting position.

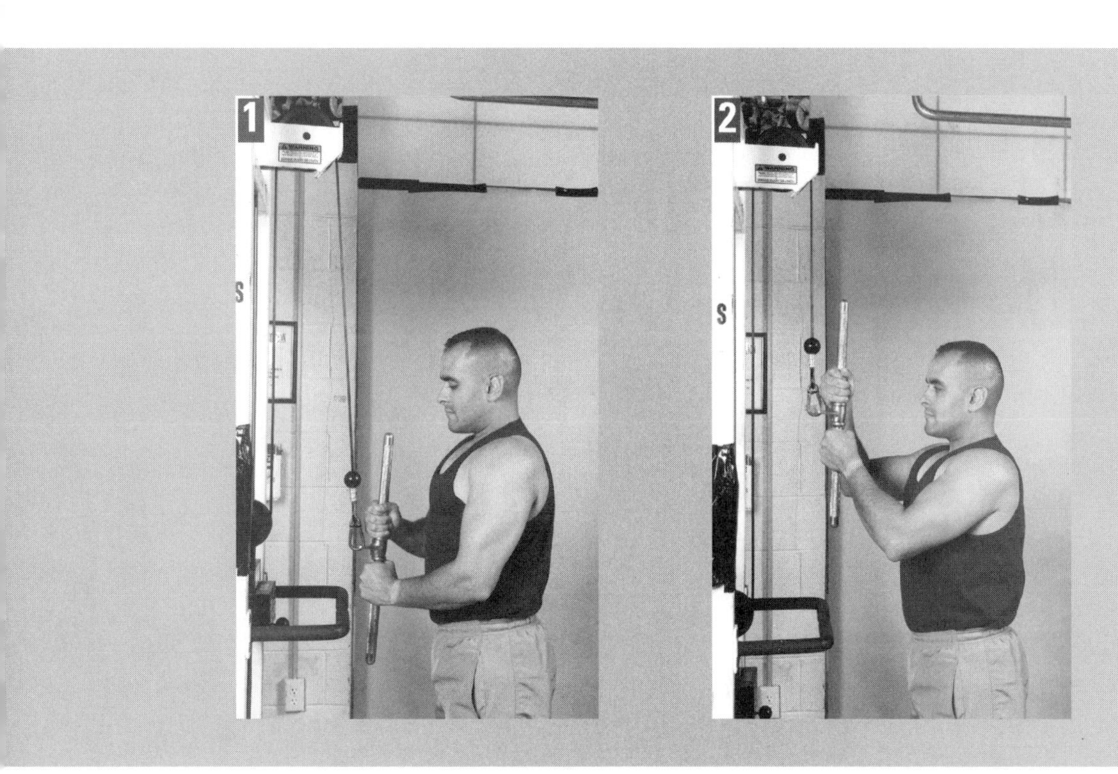

10. Dynaband Side Bend

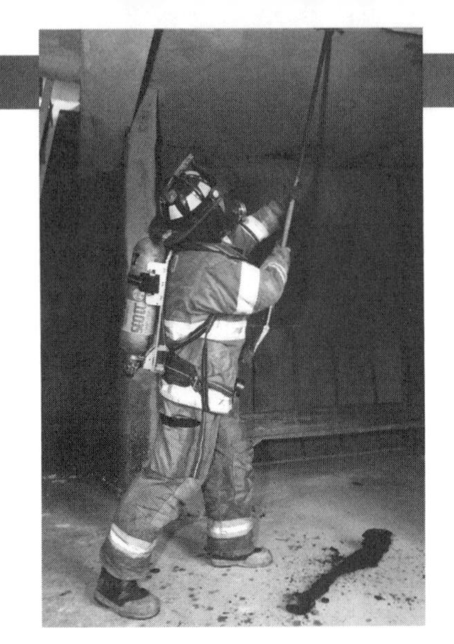

Imagine that you're pulling down some sections of an upper wall or ceiling to inspect for extension of fire.

Target: Obliques

Starting Position: Tie the resistance band to an immovable object so that the band is at the highest point your arms can reach. Stand with your feet about shoulder-width apart and the resistance band to the side. Grasp the band and stand tall.

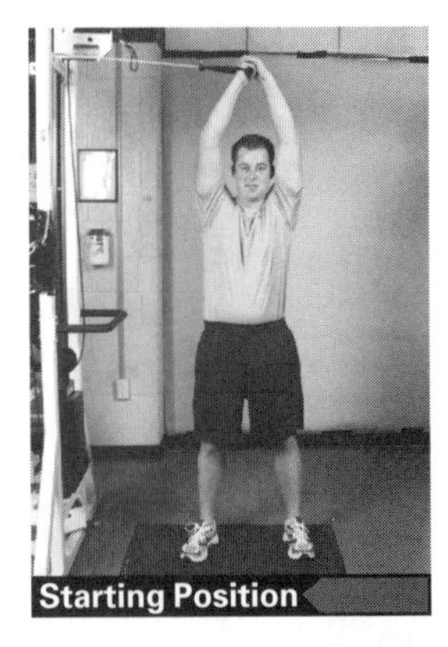
Starting Position

1. Bend at the waist, away from the object.
2. Slowly return to starting position and then repeat to the other side.

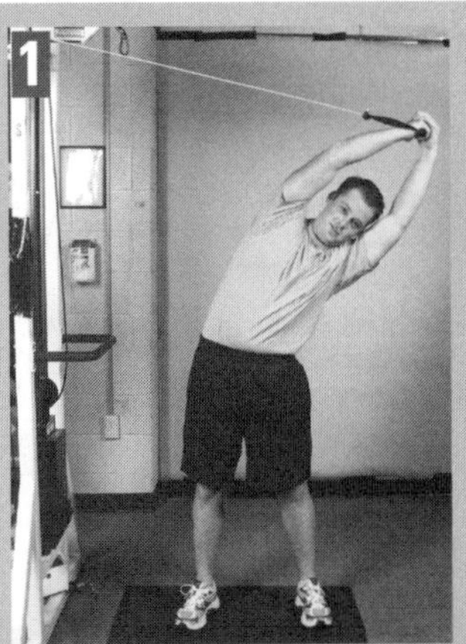

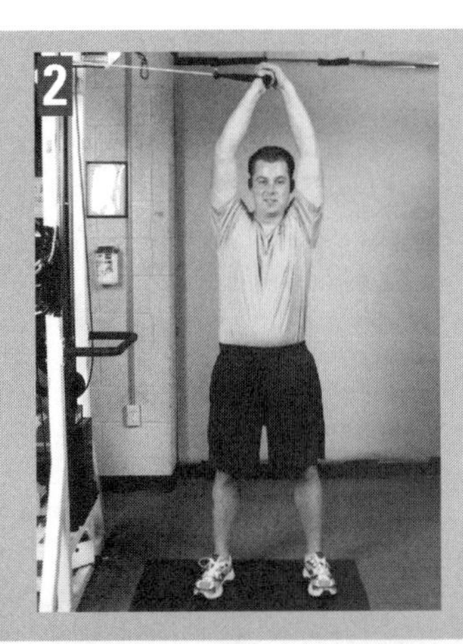

Alternative: Cable Side Bend

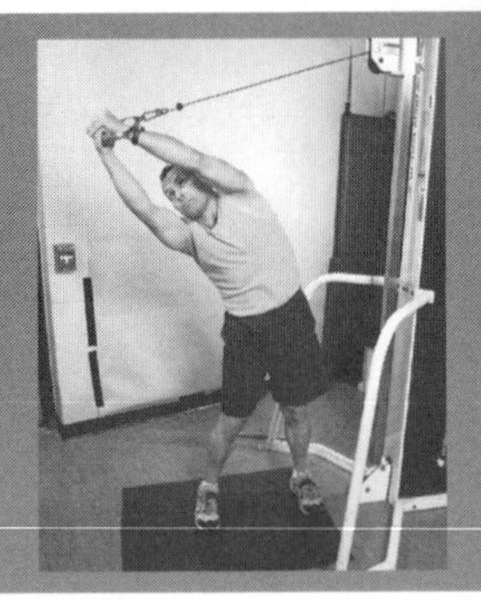

FIREFIGHTER CANDIDATE'S WORKOUT

Recognizing the need to develop a physical ability test that could fairly and accurately measure the job-oriented physical capacities of firefighter candidates in the United States and Canada, the International Association of Fire Chiefs (IAFC) and International Association of Fire Fighters (IAFF) partnered with ten career fire departments in 1996 to develop a universal Candidate Physical Ability Test (CPAT) for firefighters. The CPAT was actually just one important component of a much-larger initiative designed wholeheartedly to improve the health, safety and performance of firefighters. To the benefit of so many firefighters today, the Joint Labor Management Wellness-Fitness Initiative has been adopted and is utilized by fire departments across the continent.

The CPAT is composed of eight basic yet crucial firefighting tasks. The tasks are completed one right after the other in a pre-set order. The entire sequence of tasks must be successfully completed within 10 minutes and 20 seconds time. Candidates are required to wear long pants, a shirt, sneakers or shoes, gloves, a strapped hardhat and a 50-pound weighted vest throughout the test. The vest is intended to simulate the weight of protective clothing and equipment worn by working firefighters. During the stair-climbing event, an additional 25 pounds must be worn on the shoulders of the vest. This is done to mimic the added weight of heavy tools and equipment typically carried by firefighters, especially at high-rise-building fire operations.

The following are the eight CPAT tasks:

1. **Stair Climb:** Wearing an additional 12.5-pound weight on each shoulder, the candidate walks on the StepMill without use of the handrail. The candidate walks on the StepMill for 20 seconds at a pace of 50 steps per second and then immediately thereafter (without any break) for an additional three minutes at a pace of 60 steps per minute. This task simulates a firefighter ascending stairs at a fire operation.
2. **Hose Drag:** The candidate walks or runs, dragging a length of empty hose 75 feet. The candidate then makes a 90-degree turn to the right and continues for another 25 feet to a designated boxed-out area. Once inside the designated area, the candidate kneels down on one or both knees and pulls the remainder of the lead 50-foot length of hose into the box. This event simulates the dragging and pulling of a hose line into position for the extinguishment of fire.
3. **Equipment Carry:** The candidate lifts two saws of approximately 28–32 pounds each

from a tool cabinet one at a time and places them on the ground. Picking up one saw in each hand, the candidate then walks 75 feet out around a cone, and 75 feet back to the tool box. Both saws are placed on the ground and then one at a time lifted and placed back into the tool box. This event simulates the removal, transport and replacement of power saws on a fire apparatus at a fire or emergency operation.

4. **Ladder Raise and Extension:** The candidate walks over to a ladder that is lying on the ground. Grabbing a hold of the ladder's top rung, the candidate raises the top of the ladder over his or her head. Grabbing and pushing upward on each rung as he or she proceeds forward, the candidate moves forward, raising the ladder to an upright position. Next, the candidate walks over to a vertically secured 24-foot extension ladder, grabs a hold of the ladder rope (halyard) and pulls it downward in a hand-over-hand fashion to fully extend the ladder. This is done from within a designated area (box) marked on the floor. These tasks mimic the raising and extending of a portable ladder at a fire or emergency operation.
5. **Forcible Entry:** Using a 10-pound sledgehammer, the candidate repeatedly strikes the designated target until sufficient cumulative force has been applied, sounding an alarm. This activity replicates the action of forcing open a locked door at a fire operation.
6. **Search:** The candidate crawls through a darkened maze. This event intends to simulate the actions taken by a firefighter crawling around and searching for victims or fire at a fire or emergency operation.
7. **Rescue:** Grabbing a 165-pound mannequin by its harness handles, the candidate drags the mannequin 35 feet out around a drum, and back another 35 feet to the finish line. This action mimics the removal of a victim at a fire or emergency operation.
8. **Ceiling Breach and Pull:** The candidate takes a hold of the six-foot pike pole provided, places the pike pole tip up into the marked area on a small weighted door at ceiling level and pushes the hinged door completely up three times. The candidate then uses the pike pole to hook onto a hanging weighted ceiling device and pulls the device completely down five times. The candidate completes four sets of three pushing and five pulling movements. This activity simulates the actions that a firefighter must take with the use of a six-foot pike pole at a fire operation to examine a ceiling for fire extension.

The Firefighter Candidate's Workout is designed to develop the specific strengths necessary to successfully complete the CPAT. Special exercises focus on the muscles primarily involved in the performance of each test task. To further accelerate training improvement and gains, the selected exercises have been sequenced in the same order as the corresponding test tasks.

Given that the majority of test tasks require a relatively high number of repetitions to complete, we recommend that you emphasize the development of muscular endurance in your training. Working between 8–12 repetitions through the set will certainly improve necessary power and strength. However, completing 15–20 repetitions at least twice a week is probably even more important and therefore advisable.

With the calisthenic exercises, challenge yourself and push to the point of fatigue. However, *never* strain or otherwise compromise your form to squeeze out that one last rep. It's not worth the risk of injury. As with the other programs, we recommend that you begin with just one set and build as you gain strength and muscular endurance.

To be truly successful with this challenging physical ability test, you definitely need to be well-trained aerobically. Develop a gradual and progressive aerobic training program that best supports your CPAT training efforts. A StepMill, where available, is clearly the exercise tool of choice. Prospective firefighters that we routinely work with build through a training progression on the StepMill that ultimately leads to the use of a 50-pound (or greater) vest. Experience has shown that in order for candidates to be successful with this test, they must be well-enough aerobically conditioned to dismount the StepMill during the test feeling like it was a warm-up rather than a death-defying feat. If you're beat up or exhausted upon completion of the Stair Climb event, your chances for success are remote.

We recommend that you develop a personal conditioning program that involves participation in both the Firefighter Candidate's Workout and a progressive aerobic training routine. Try to build to the point where you complete the Firefighter Candidate's Workout three times a week and train aerobically almost everyday. Although training on the StepMill with a weighted vest would be most productive, you can also use a few flights of stairs. Finally, if provided, you should take advantage of every opportunity to train on the CPAT course or perform each of the actual tasks from the CPAT events. This will help you to identify your physical strengths and weakness and give you a very good idea of what you need to emphasize in terms of training. Once you've sufficiently developed your fitness, completing training runs through the CPAT course will enable you to pick up on any of the finer details involved with your actions and to refine your overall task performance. If you've done your homework and trained consistently, tough and intelligently, this final phase of training should serve as the icing on the cake.

1. Machine Stepping

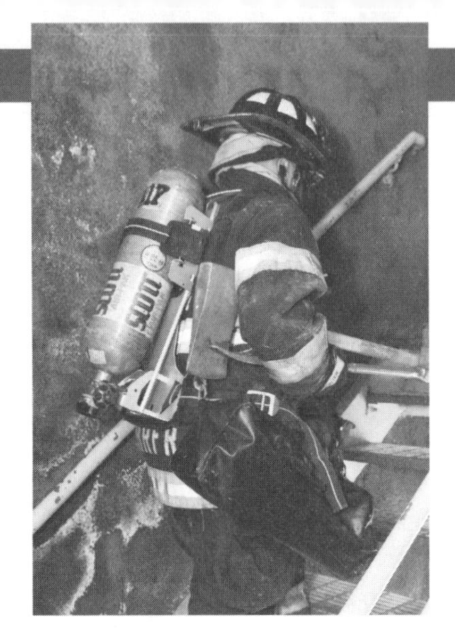

Target: Quadriceps, gluteals

Position: Step onto the machine and follow the screened programming messages to begin. Step at a cadence of 1 step per second. Lean slightly and look straight ahead to maintain an upright posture.

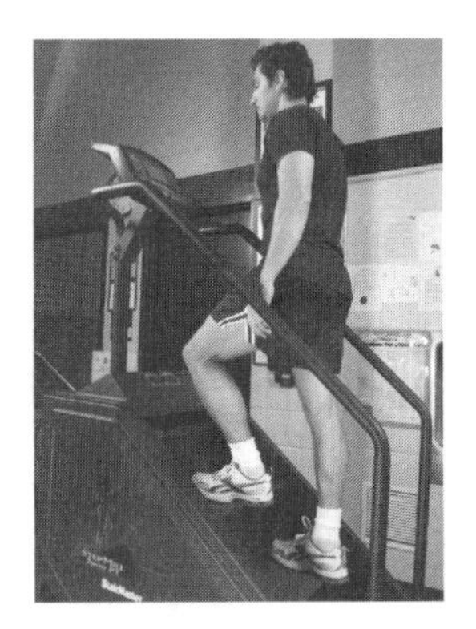

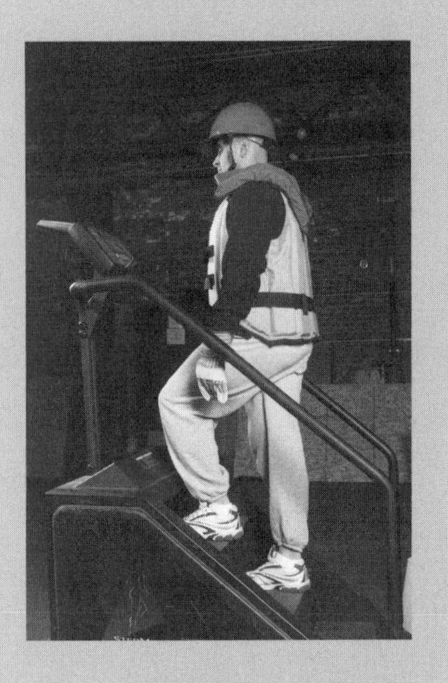

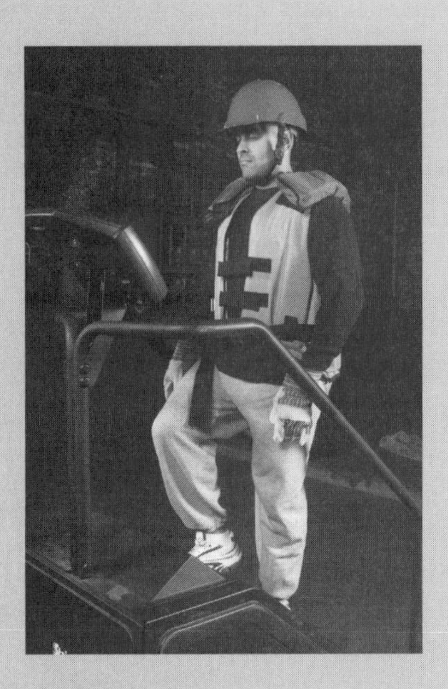

2. Dumbbell One-Arm Row

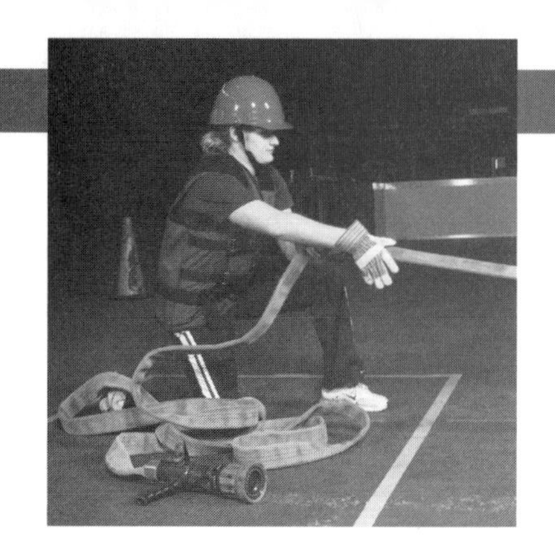

Target: Latissimus dorsi, teres major, posterior deltoid, rhomboids, trapezuis, biceps

Starting Position: Bend over and place one hand on a chair. Hold the weight with the other hand and let it hang to the ground. Keep your knees bent and your back straight.

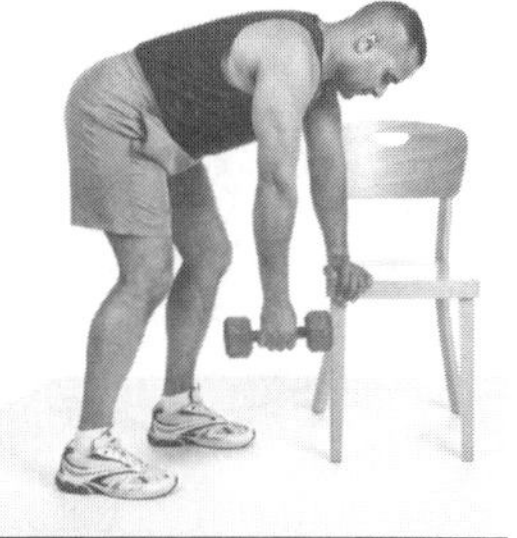

Starting Position

1. Leading with your elbow, lift the weight straight up and hold.
2. Slowly return to starting position.

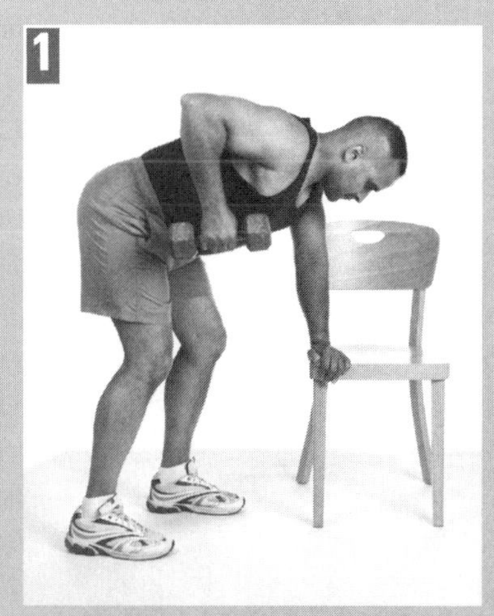

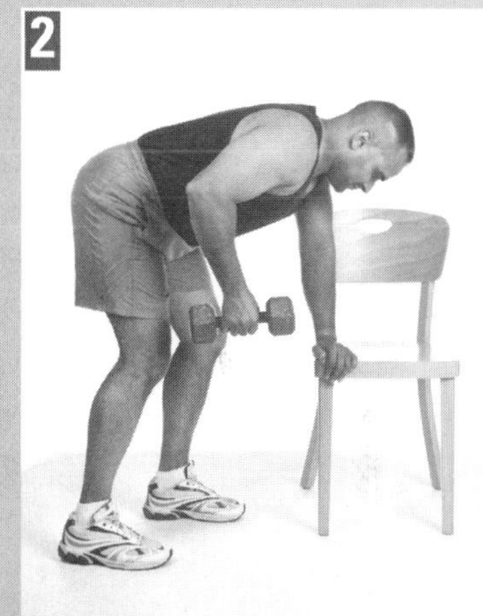

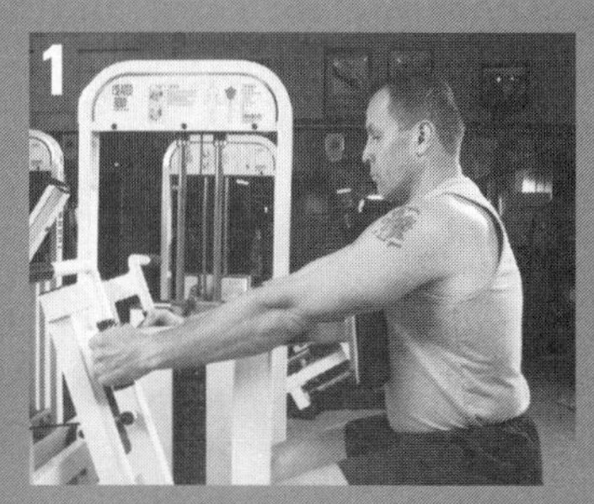

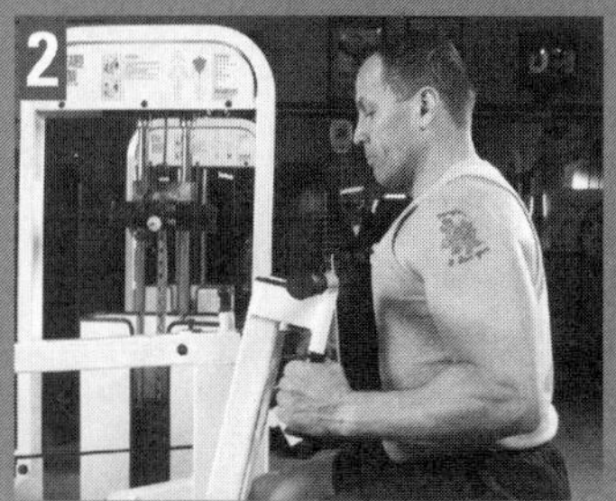

Alternative: Machine Compound Row

1. Sit facing the machine. Set the seat height so that the chest pad is at mid-chest level and your hands can just grab the vertical handles.
2. Pull the handles backward as far as possible and hold. Slowly return to starting position.

3. Dumbbell Upright Row

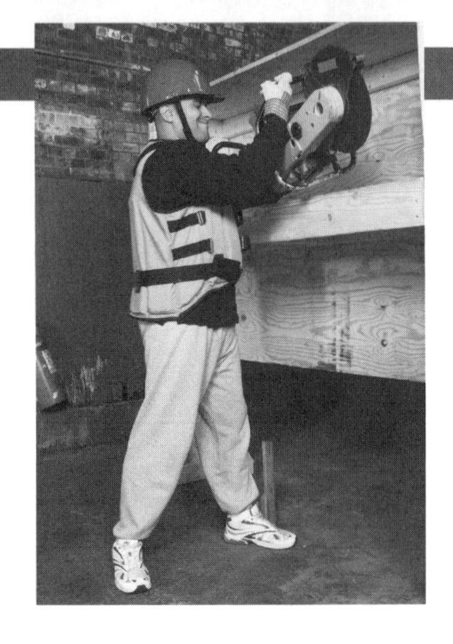

Target: Lateral deltoids

Starting Position: Stand with your feet about shoulder-width apart, holding the weights with your arms fully extended.

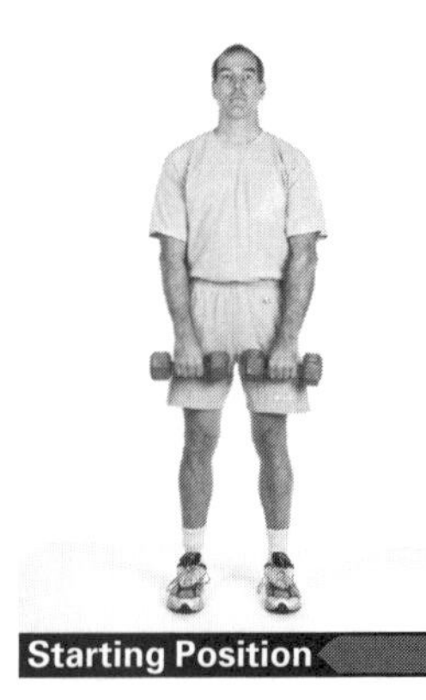

Starting Position

1. Pull the weights straight up to the fronts of your shoulders, keeping your elbows above the weights. Hold.
2. Slowly return to starting position.

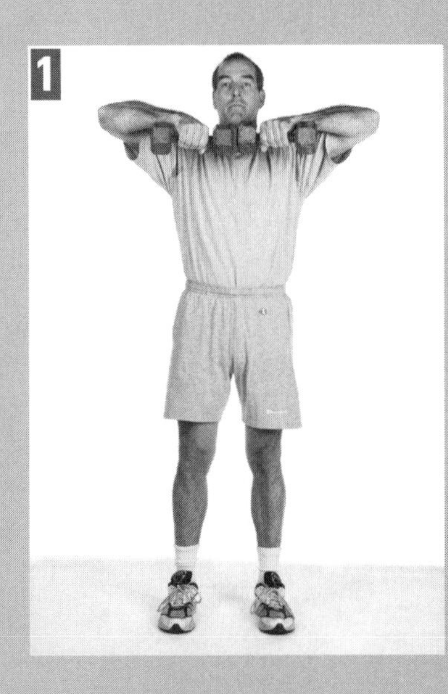

1

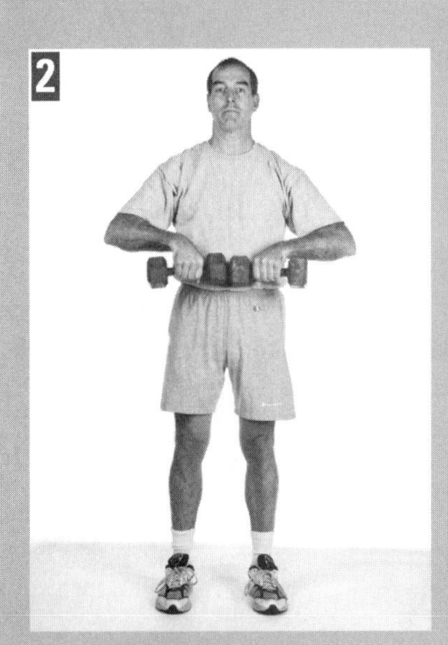

2

4. Dumbbell Curl & Press

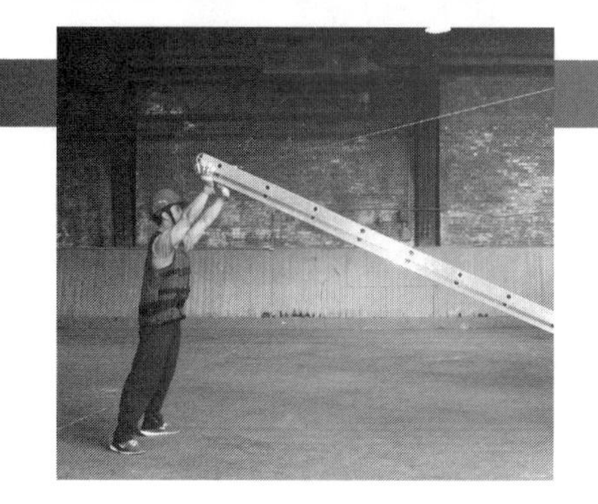

Target: Anterior deltoid, brachialis, triceps

Starting Position: Stand with your feet about shoulder-width apart, holding the weights at your sides, palms facing inward.

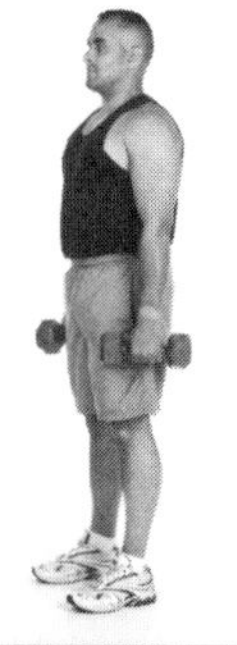

Starting Position

1. Bend your elbows to curl the weights to your shoulders.
2. Then press the weights overhead until your arms are almost fully extended. Hold.
3. Slowly return to starting position.

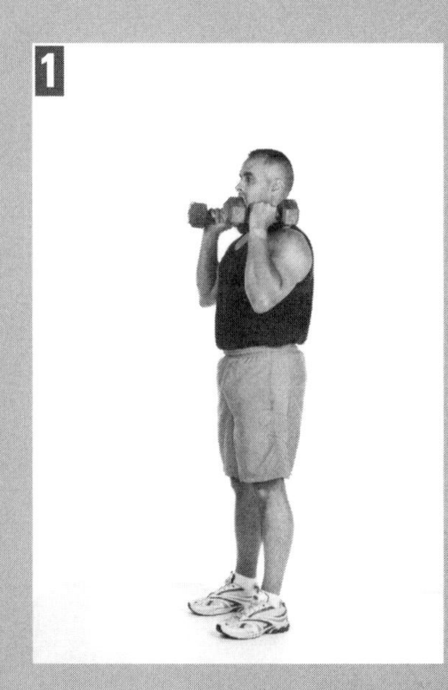

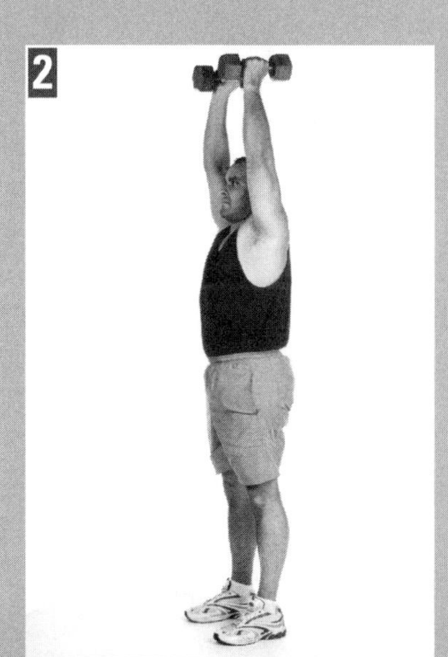

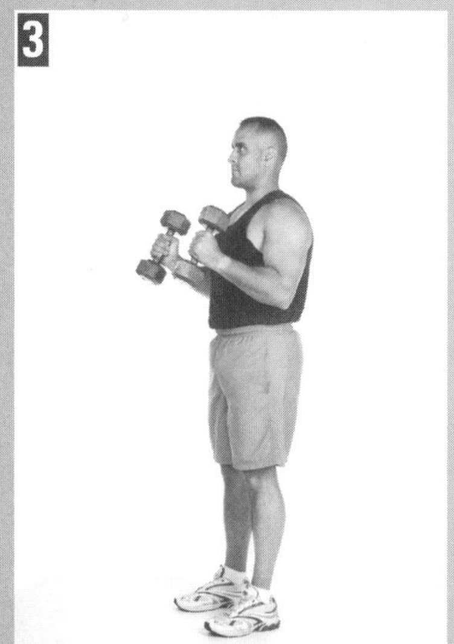

5. Dynaband Swing

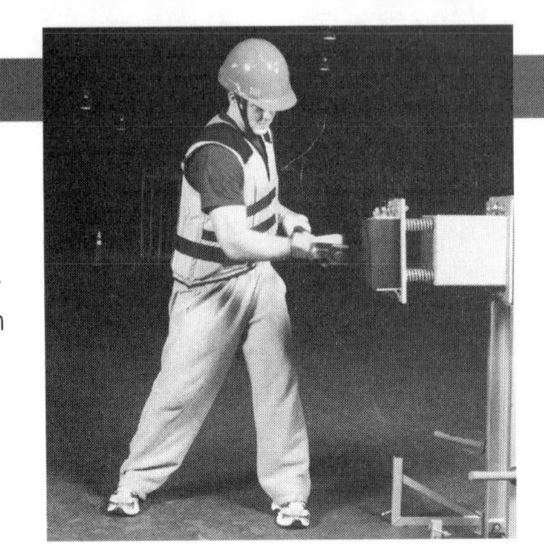

Target: Obliques, tranverse abdominis

Starting Position: Tie the resistance band to an immovable object at a height between waist and chest level. Stand with your feet about shoulder-width apart and the resistance band to the side. Grasp the band with both hands. Take one step away to make sure the band is taut.

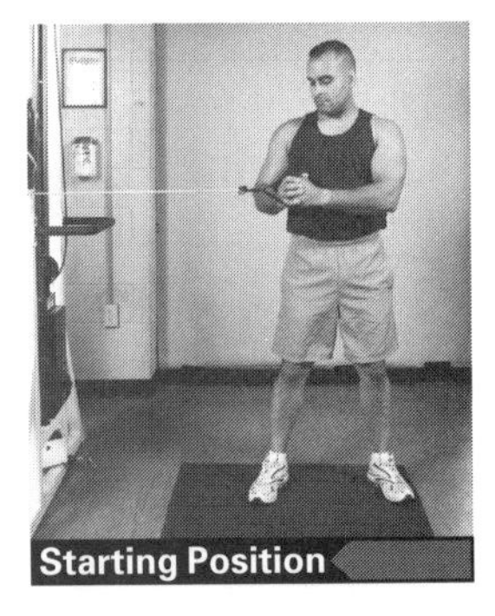
Starting Position

1. Turn your hips and trunk away from the immovable object. Hold.
2. Slowly return to starting position.

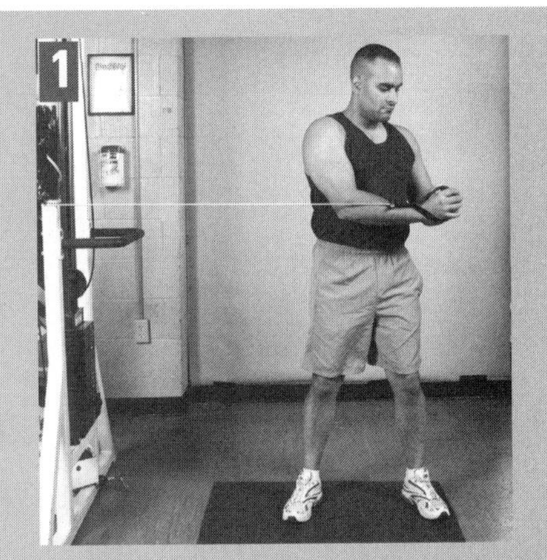
1

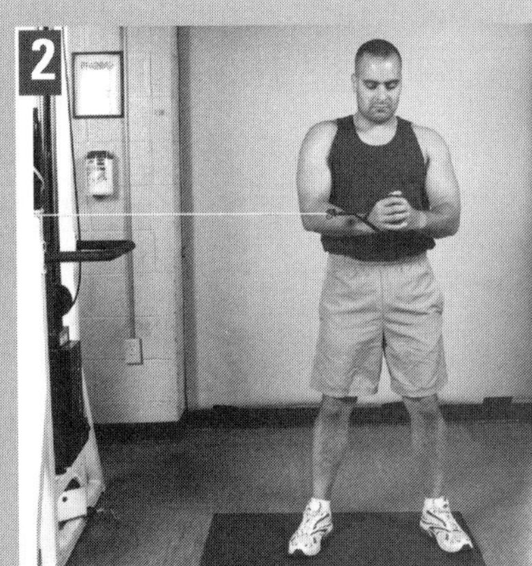
2

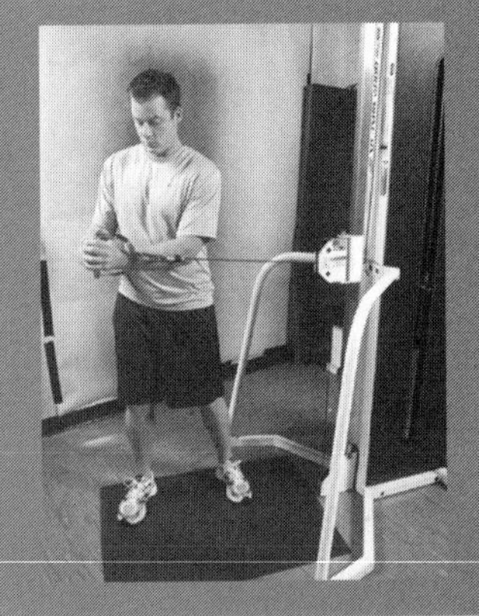

Alternative: Cable Swing

6. Cable Rope Pull-Down

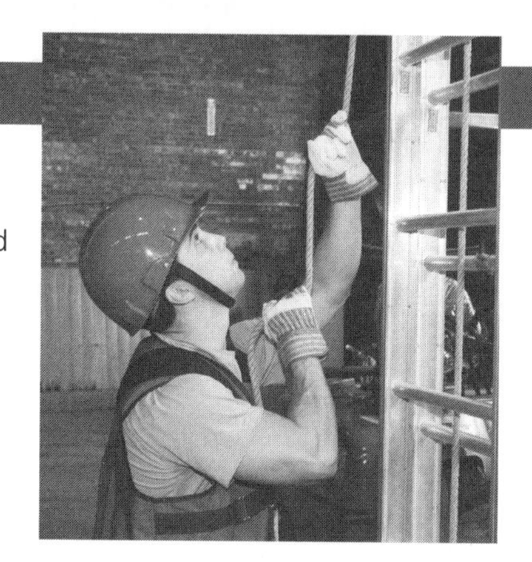

Target: Latissimus dorsi, biceps

Starting Position: Sit facing the machine. Grasp the rope with one hand above the other, palms facing away, making sure your arms are almost fully extended.

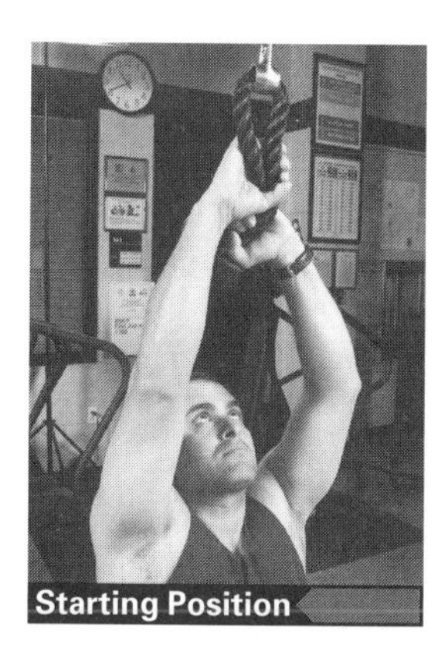
Starting Position

1. Pull downward on the rope, using your upper hand to do most of the work. Hold.

2. Slowly return to starting position and then repeat the exercise, emphasizing the use of your other hand.

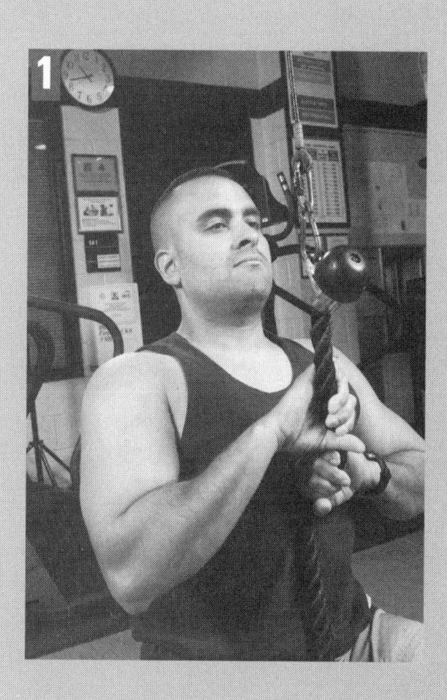
1

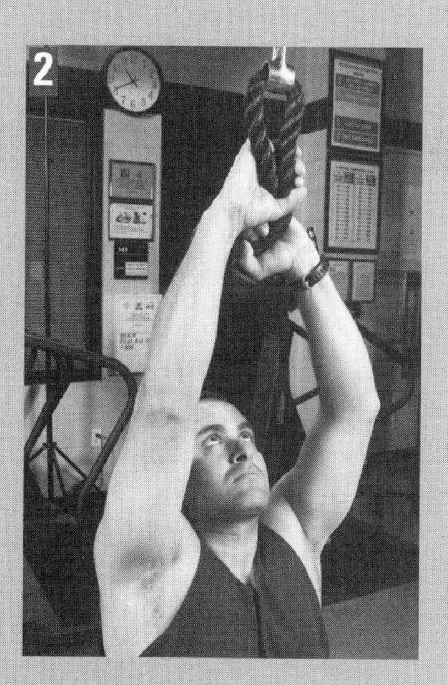
2

7. Back Extension

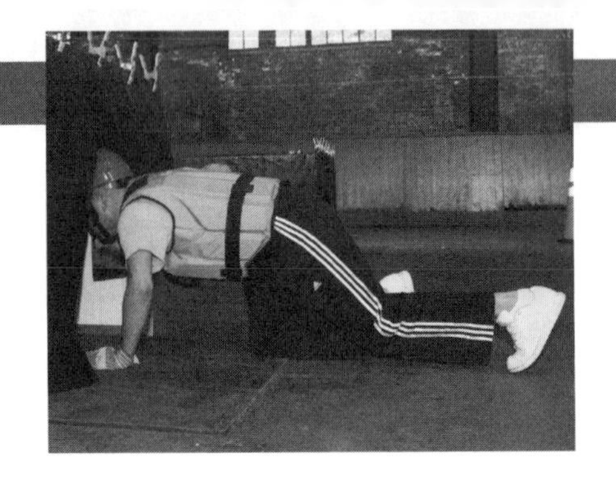

Target: Spinal erectors

Starting Position: Lie face down on the ground. Stack your hands on the floor and rest your chin on them.

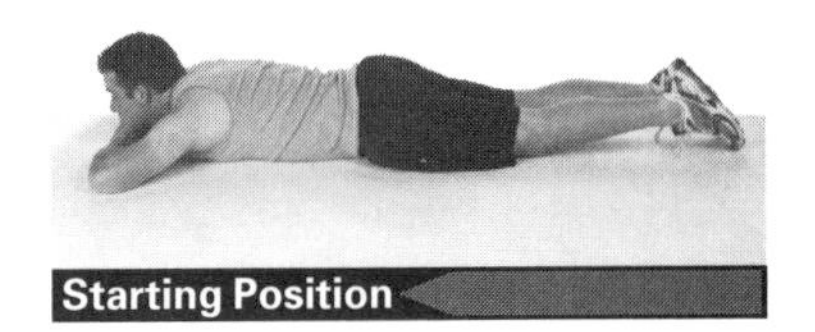

Starting Position

1. Slowly raise your arms and legs off the ground a few inches and hold.
2. Slowly return to starting position.

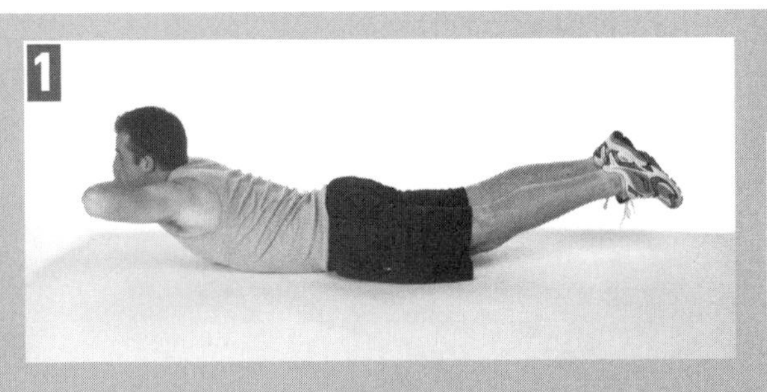

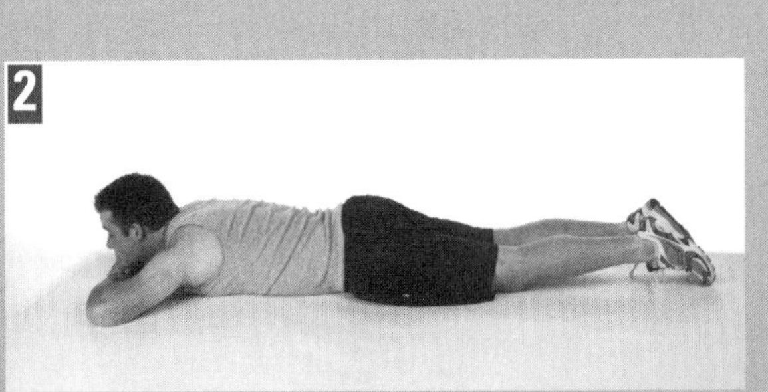

Alternative: Roman Chair—Back Extension

1. Lie face down and place your thighs on the large pad and your ankles under the support pads.
2. Bend at the waist and lower your body toward the floor. Raise and extend your waist and slowly return to starting position.

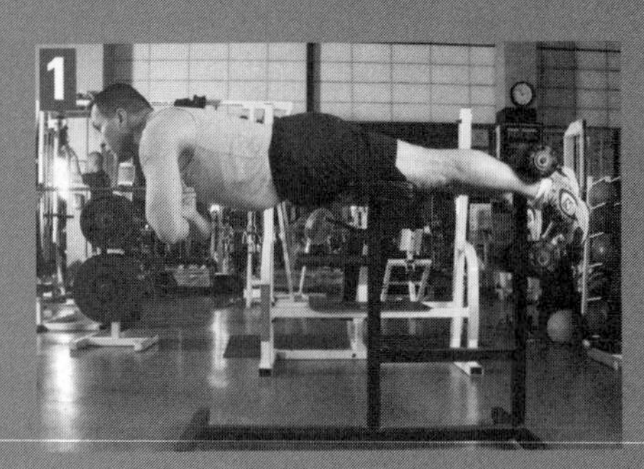

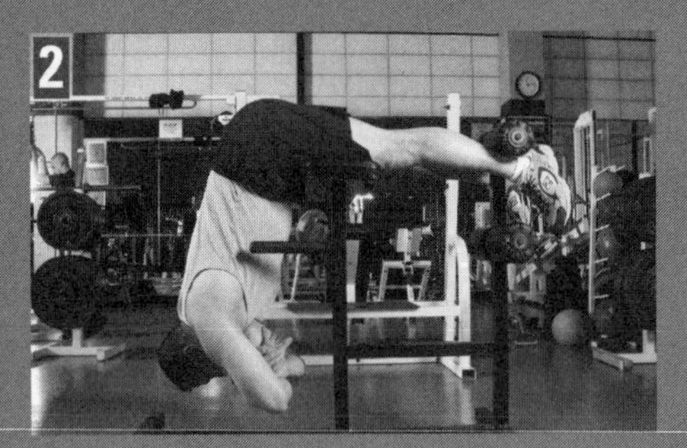

8. Diagonal Incline Crunch

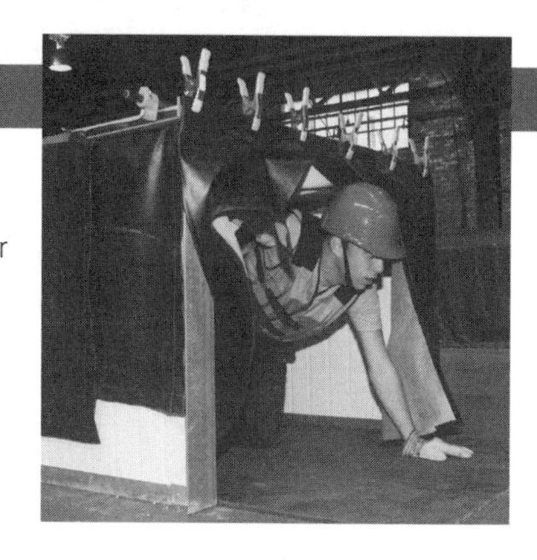

Target: Obliques, lower abdominals

Starting Position: Lie on an incline board with your hips bent and your feet hooked under the brace for support. Your shoulders should be in contact with the pad of the board.

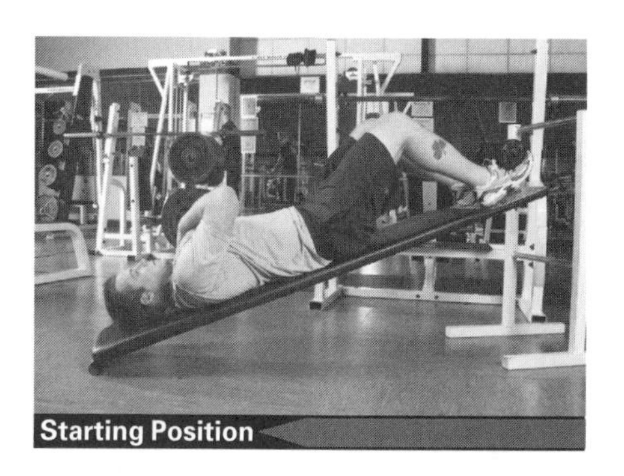
Starting Position

1. Curl your waist to raise your upper torso from the bench, moving your armpit to the opposite knee. Hold at the top.
2. Slowly return to starting position.

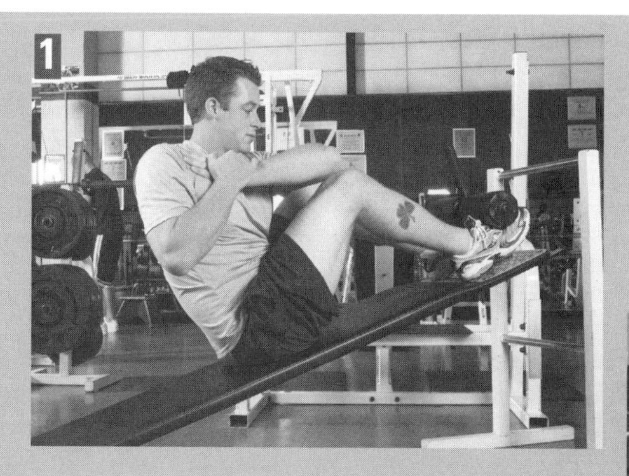
1

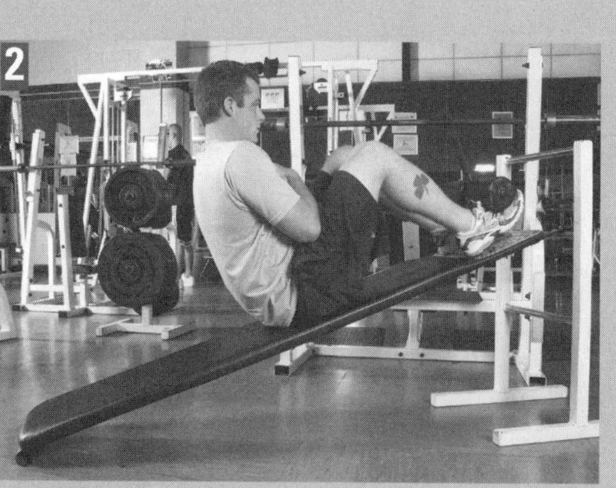
2

9. Dumbbell One-Arm Row

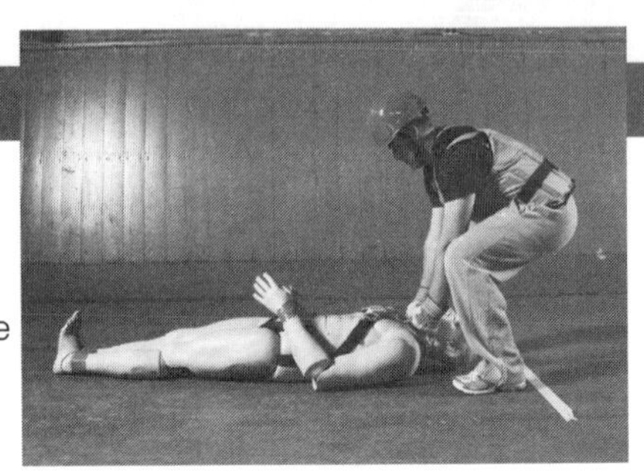

Target: Latissimus dorsi, teres major, posterior deltoid, rhomboids, trapezuis, biceps

Starting Position: Bend over and place one hand on a chair. Hold the weight with the other hand and let it hang to the ground. Keep your knees bent and your back straight.

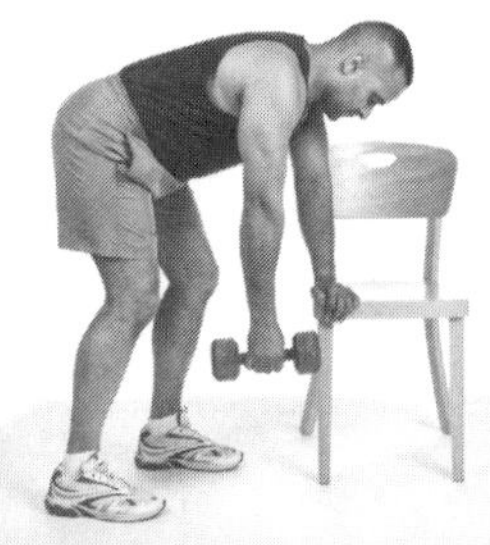

Starting Position

1 Leading with your elbow, lift the weight straight up and hold.

2 Slowly return to starting position.

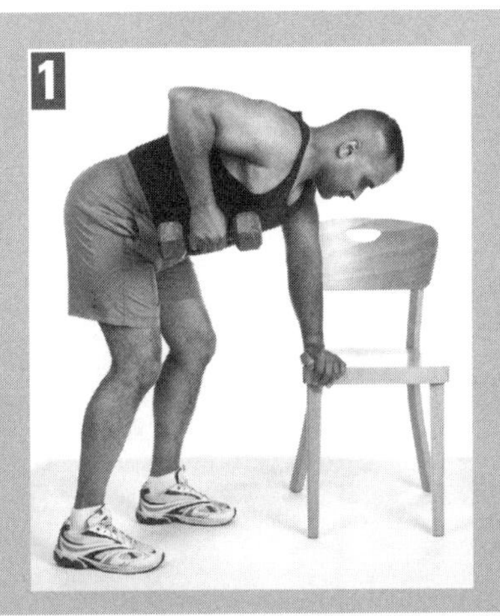

1

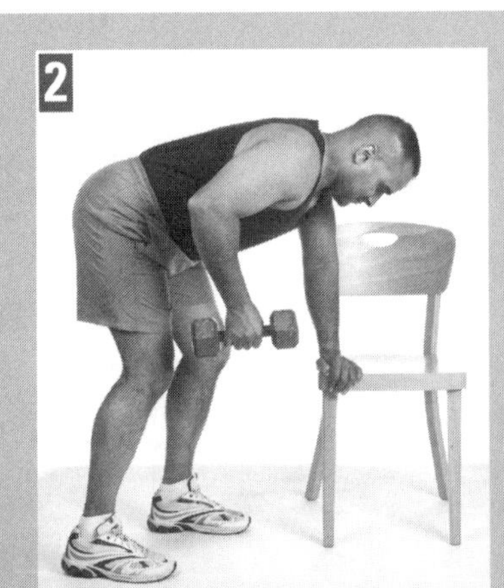

2

Alternative: Cable Low Row

1 Sit facing the machine so that your legs are extended but still slightly bent. Grab the handles, making sure your arms are completely straight.

2 Pull the handles backward as far as possible and hold. Slowly return to starting position.

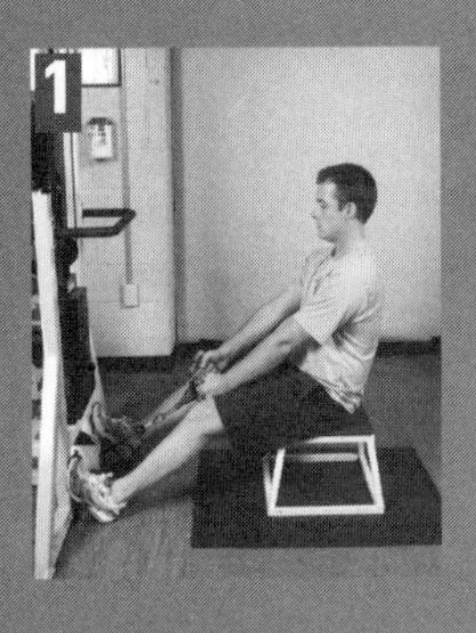

1

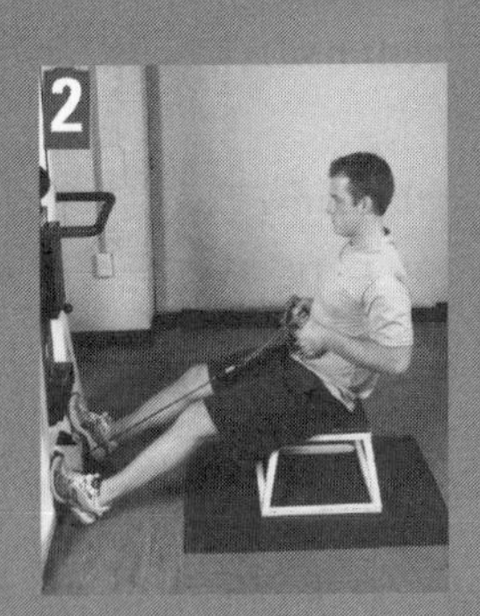

2

10. Dumbbell Squat

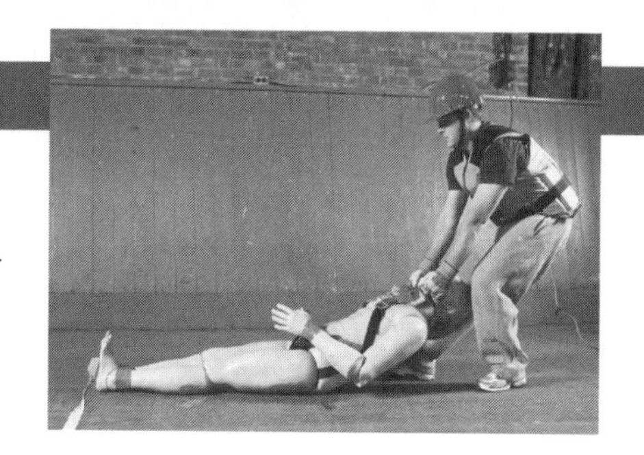

Target: Quadriceps, gastrocnemius

Starting Position: Stand with your feet slightly wider than shoulder-width apart, holding the hand weights at your sides.

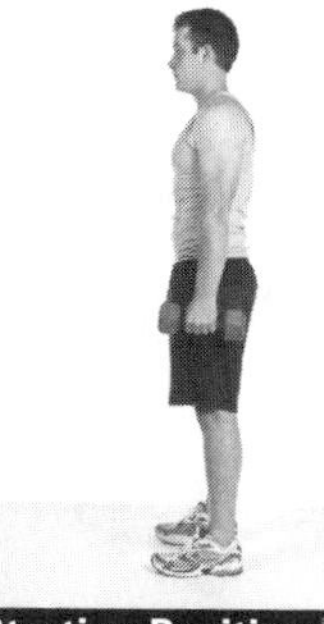

Starting Position

1 Bend your knees, moving into a sitting position, and hold.

2 Slowly return to starting position.

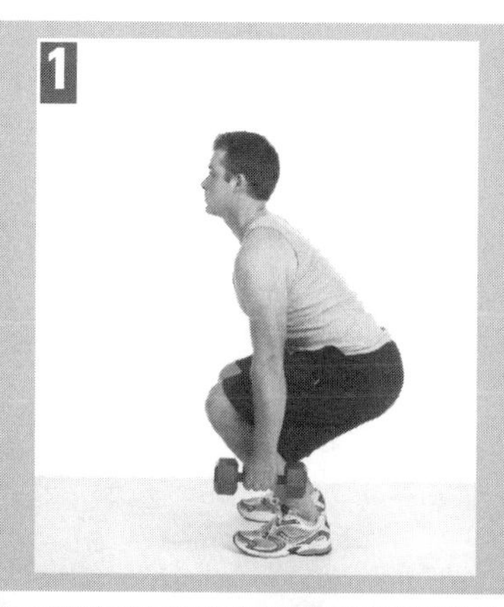

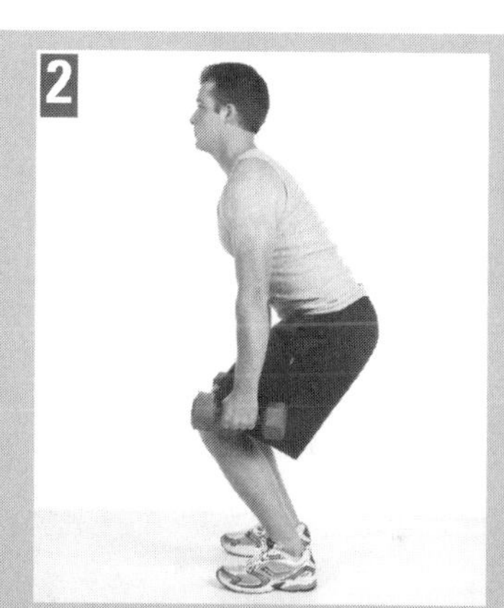

Alternative: Machine Leg Press

1 Lie down and press your lower back against the support pad. Place your feet about shoulder-width apart on the footplate. Turn the locks out of the way and grasp the handles. Bend your knees toward your chest.

2 Slowly extend your legs. Hold. Slowly return to starting position.

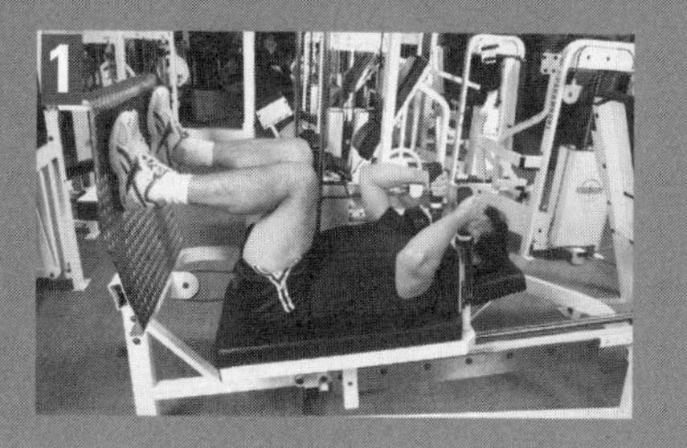

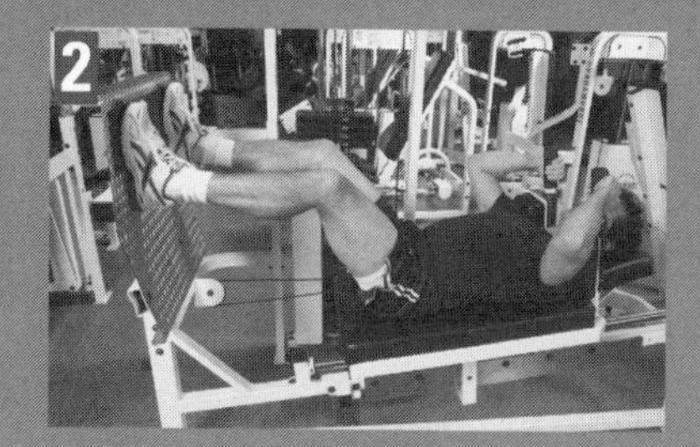

11. Combined Dumbbell Press

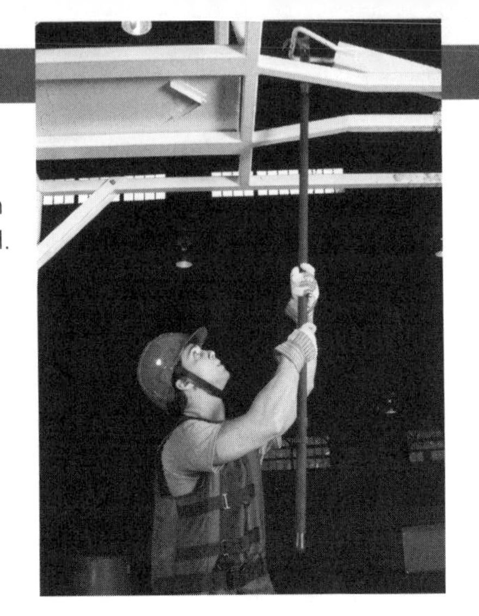

Target: Deltoids, triceps

Starting Position: Stand with your feet staggered about shoulder-width apart. Stack the weights vertically (one on top of the other) at chest level.

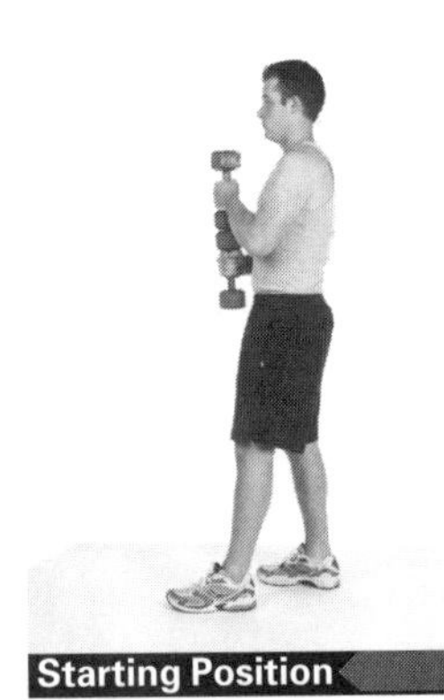
Starting Position

1. Press straight upward until your arms are almost fully extended and hold.
2. Slowly return to starting position.

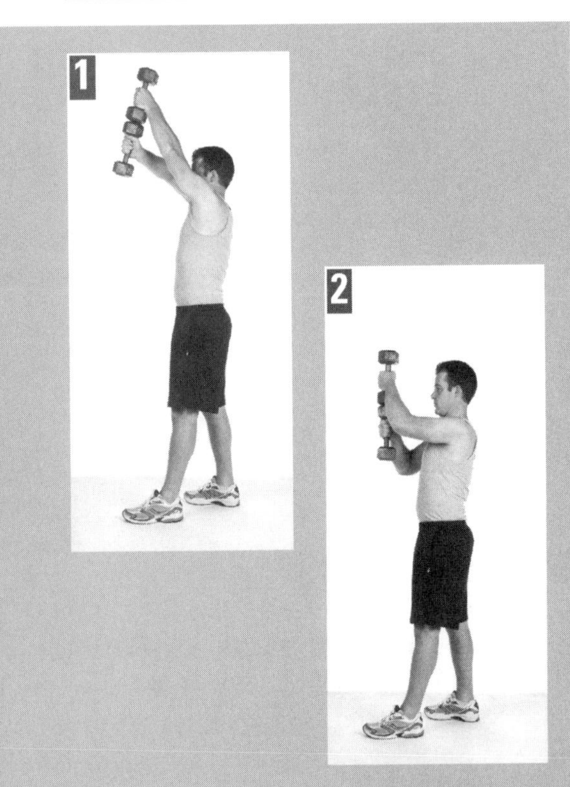

Alternative: Cable Lift & Press (Vertical Bar)

1. Stand facing the cable machine with the cable at the "low" position. Hold the straight curl bar in a vertical position with your arms slightly bent.
2. Press the bar up toward the ceiling. Slowly return to starting position.

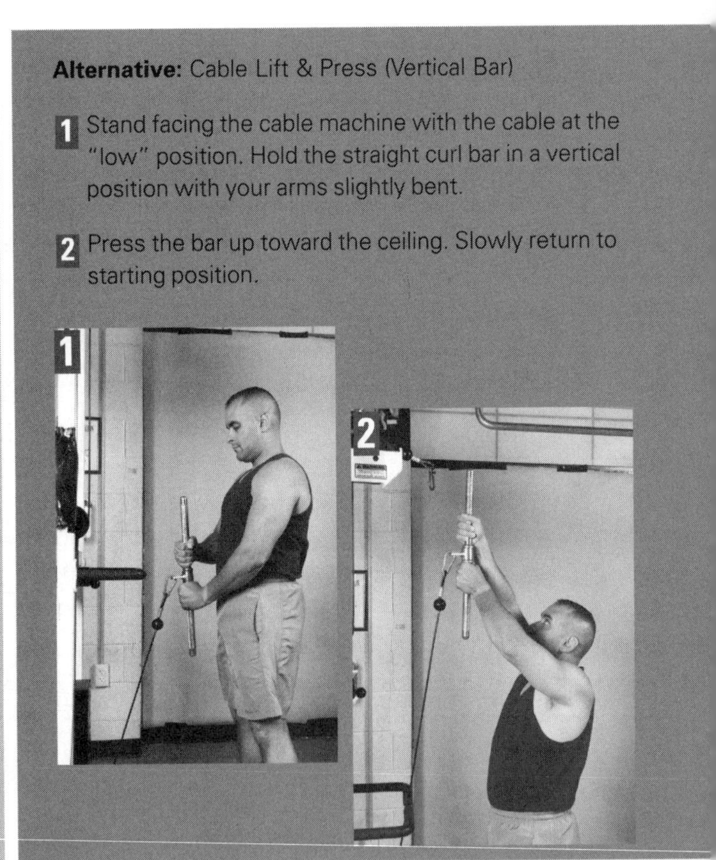

12. Cable Pull-Down (Vertical Bar)

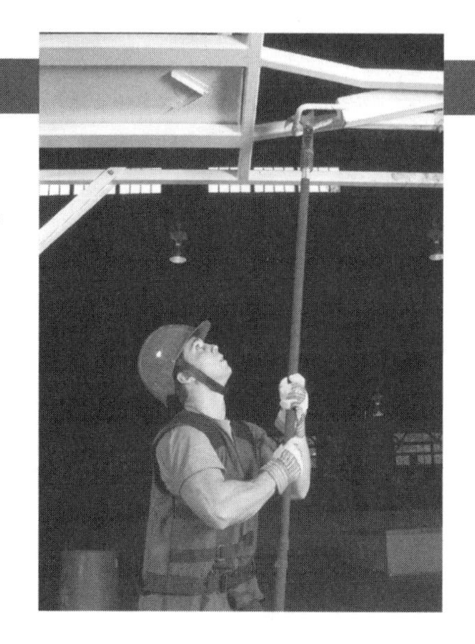

Target: Latissimus dorsi, biceps

Starting Position: Stand facing the cable machine with the cable at the "high" position. Hold the straight curl bar in a vertical position with your arms slightly bent.

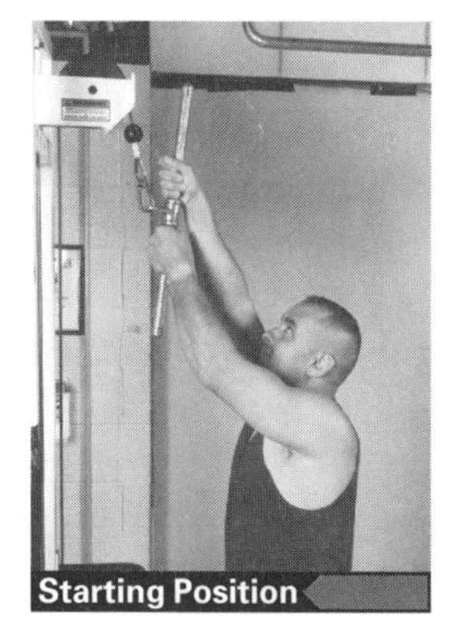
Starting Position

1. Pull the bar down toward your mid-section.
2. Slowly return to starting position.

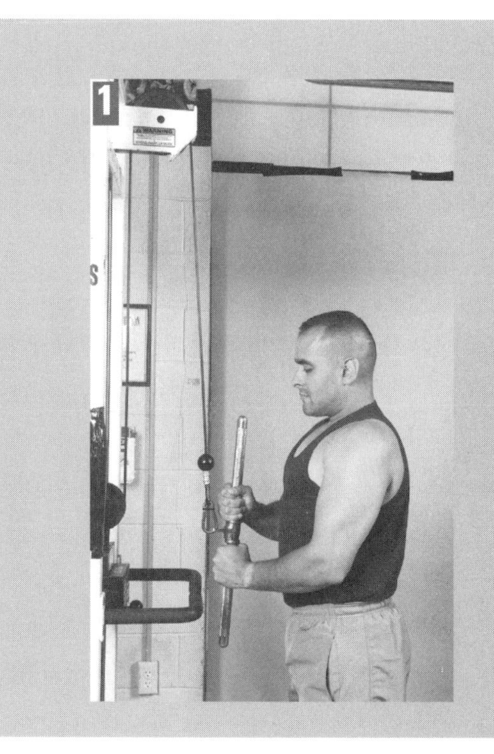

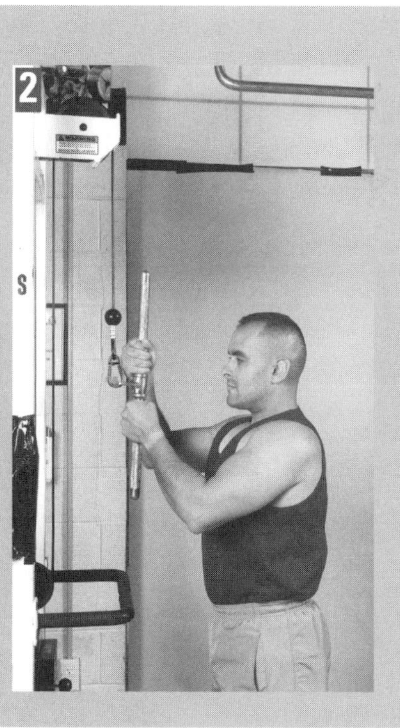

Alternate Physical Training Programs

In an effort to provide you with some interesting and productive options with your training, we've included a varied selection of alternative physical training programs specifically designed to better meet your personal training needs and interests. Consider your individual capabilities, desired goals and allotted time. Then review the programs and select the one(s) that is/are right for you.

Once you've chosen a program that seems like a good fit, refer to the given page numbers to obtain the specific instructions for each exercise movement. Then set yourself up and give it a try. Move through the exercise set at your own pace and complete the number of repetitions for each exercise that promotes the type of strength development you desire. To develop muscular endurance, complete many repetitions (15–20 or more) with each exercise and move rapidly from one exercise to the next without much time for recovery. Research suggests that you may obtain some aerobic training benefit as well. To develop muscular strength, perform fewer repetitions (8–12 or less) using heavier weights and taking longer periods of recovery between exercise sets.

Remember to always be mindful of your body positions and movements when stretching and performing resistance training. Emphasize good form and lifting techniques throughout the full range of motion and *never* excessively strain for the sake of one additional rep. Train *smart,* and THEN train tough—that's the way to achieve the most rapid gains and greatest training success.

ROLL-CALL WORKOUT

This brief yet comprehensive training program is perfect for starting your day. It's great for individuals who have particularly busy daily schedules and for firefighters who'd like to get in a good physical warm-up just prior to their tour of duty. The Roll-Call Workout begins with a set of four important stretching exercises. These exercises involve six different movements that provide a nice, brief general-body warm-up and stretch. As usual, the routine starts in the lower body and progresses upward. This should make it very easy to remember and relatively simple to complete. The six strength-training exercises follow the same pattern of progressively moving from the lower to upper body. All of the exercises are calisthenics, which allow you to complete the program quickly and easily in almost any location: the fire house, a hotel room or your living room. If you'd like to further challenge yourself on a given day, you always have the option of completing additional sets of the calisthenic exercises.

ROLL-CALL WORKOUT

PAGE	NO.	TYPE	EXERCISE
42	1	S	Motor Pump Operator Stretches
46	2	S	Controlman's Stretch
43	3	S	Roofman's Stretch
45	4	S	Outside Vent Man's Reach & Twist
71	5	C	Dumbbell Heel Raise
72	6	C	Dumbbell Lunge
75	7	C	Back Extension
74	8	C	Crunch
76	9	C	Push-Up
129	10	C	Pull-Up

S = Stretch / C = Calisthenic

SPECIAL OPERATIONS SQUAD UNIT WORKOUT

Special Operations Squad Units respond to fires and emergency incidents throughout the entire fire district in most fire departments. When you report in to the chief officer at an operation, you're expected to be prepared to perform whatever fire or emergency task that needs to get done. Consequently, you have to be sufficiently trained, experienced and physically conditioned to perform the full spectrum of engine, ladder and special operations tasks. Additionally, special operations units are often called upon to respond directly from one operation to another. The members must therefore be able to recover quickly and endure repeated demands.

This specialized training program is designed to develop your capacities to perform at the highest level. It's a very challenging program that can dramatically improve physical ability and performance on the athletic field or fireground. Given the intense nature of this workout, emphasize the maintenance of proper training balance, providing muscles and other tissues with the rest necessary between training sessions to allow for recovery and productive development.

"Firefighting is a push me—pull me occupation."[12] Whether you're forcing open a door, pulling down a ceiling, operating a nozzle or rescuing a victim, the task is likely to be physically demanding and involve either a pushing or pulling movement. This focused, high-intensity workout is designed to develop great strength and muscle size in the chest, back, shoulders and arms. It's the perfect program for individuals who want to develop peak strength in the upper body and arms for a competitive edge in athletic competition, improved firefighting capacity and/or dynamic physical appearance. All of the upper body areas, employed extensively in the performance of engine, ladder and special operations unit tasks, are rigorously challenged. This is an outstanding arm and upper body workout for anyone looking to get in top shape, particularly high-intensity firefighters.

Three proven approaches to strength training are utilized in this training program to optimize strength and performance gains: "multi-joint to single-joint," "large to small" and "supersets." The multi-joint-to-single-joint series begins with multi-joint exercises and leads to single-joint exercises. The large-to-small series progresses from the use of greater to lesser muscle mass. Supersets are a multiple-set system of resistance training in which a series of exercises is used to develop the opposing muscle groups of one specific body part; the exercise series alternates the use of opposing muscle groups. Used together, these methods promote rapid development of the primary muscles involved in select movements, as well as the accessory muscles that provide them with assistance. Balanced training with the use of this special program is likely to result in dynamic and comprehensive muscular development.

The upper body superset is composed of six exercises to be completed in series, one right after the other; 15–20 repetitions are executed with each exercise in the first set. To obtain the full benefit of this training method, you shouldn't take any break for recovery between exercises. And, as soon as you've completed the final (sixth) exercise of the set, you should move immediately back to the first exercise and begin your next set. Continue using the same weight for all three sets—only the number of repetitions changes. After completing 15–20 repetitions of the first set, you should complete 8–12 in the second and 3–5 in the third.

The Special Operations Squad Unit Workout is an extremely taxing program specifically designed for the peak development of high-performance athletes and firefighters. If used properly, this premier training tool can produce undeniably significant gains in upper body strength and muscular endurance. You'll see, feel and exhibit the effects of this training program in whatever field of activity you participate.

SPECIAL OPERATIONS SQUAD UNIT WORKOUT

PAGE	NO.	PRIMARY EXERCISES	PAGE	ALTERNATE EXERCISES
98	1	Dumbbell Bench Press	*not pictured*	Machine Bench Press
99	2	Cable Low Row	99	Dumbbell One-Arm Row
102	3	Cable Lift & Press (Vertical Bar)	102	Combined Dumbbell Press
103	4	Cable Pull-Down (Vertical Bar)	96	Cable Rope Pull-Down
87	5	Cable Triceps Press-Down	87	Dumbbell Kickback
79	6	Dumbbell Twisting Curl	86	Dumbbell Curl

PAGE	NO.	HOME EXERCISES
76	1	Push-Up
77	2	Dumbbell One-Arm Row
78	3	Dumbbell Overhead Press
128	4	Close-Grip Chin-Up
80	5	Dumbbell Kickback
79	6	Dumbbell Twisting Curl

SPECIAL OPERATIONS RESCUE UNIT WORKOUT

Special Operations Rescue Units respond to unique fire and emergency operations as well as to structural fires. The members of these units are highly trained in the specialized area of victim rescue. They cut people out of demolished vehicles, remove them from confined spaces and grasp them from window ledges while tethered to a rope. Whether operating hydraulic tools, removing heavy collapsed debris or clutching a victim high above the ground from a rope, Rescue Unit firefighters must be extremely fit to get the job done. They need great upper and lower body strength and, most importantly, a rock solid core. Any weakness in the abdominal, chest or back area is an open invitation to serious injury, especially in the lower back.

To expertly complete critical rescue tasks and minimize the risk of injury, Rescue Unit firefighters need to possess a powerful body core. Their need for serious conditioning in this body area is absolute. Too many firefighters find this out the hard way, generally from a physical therapist while on injured reserve. As a performance-oriented firefighter/athlete, you desire to be a player not a spectator; you want to be on the field, *not* on the bench, so be proactive, jump right into this workout and start developing your core. *Train to gain and avoid the pain.*

If you're an athlete involved in almost any type of sport or activity, your physical ability and performance depend largely upon the strength and fitness of your core. Whether you're driving a golf ball toward the green or a soft ball over the fence, the root of your power is one in the same: it's within your core. Work this program with diligence and you'll develop your personal core of power. This program is also ideal for those who aren't necessarily interested in athletic competition but are willing to push themselves a little to develop a great look and/or enjoy the sensational feeling of peak fitness.

This focused and demanding "core" program was specifically designed to enable training in whatever environment is most convenient for you. Having access to a well-equipped training facility will provide you with a greater variety of exercise options. However, by design this program can just as easily be done in the comfort and convenience of your home. All you need to do to get started are a little space, two lightweight dumbbells and a resistive exercise band (e.g., Fitstrap) that can be purchased at a medical supply store or online.

Begin by completing just one set. Work through the training routine slowly to develop a good sense of the exercise movements and the relative demands of the entire session. Once you feel comfortable completing one set, you may want to move up and add another set. That's fine, but we really encourage you *not* to rush; it's much more important to complete this program more often than more intensely. Three times a week, with a day or two of rest in between sessions, would be ideal. Remember, adequate rest is essential for the promotion of optimal development.

SPECIAL OPERATIONS RESCUE UNIT WORKOUT

PAGE	NO.	PRIMARY EXERCISES	PAGE	ALTERNATE EXERCISES
117	1	Machine Leg Press	73	Dumbbell Squat
92	2	Cable Swing	92	Dynaband Swing
98	3	Dumbbell Bench Press	*not pictured*	Machine Bench Press
84	4	Machine Compound Row	99	Cable Low Row
126	5	Twisting Cable Crunch	88	Diagonal Incline Crunch
127	6	Machine Back Extension	90	Roman Chair
89	7	Dumbbell Fly	*not pictured*	Machine Fly
104	8	Cable Side Bend	104	Dynaband Side Bend

PAGE	NO.	HOME EXERCISES
73	1	Dumbbell Squat
92	2	Dynaband Swing
76	3	Push-Up
77	4	Dumbbell One-Arm Row
88	5	Diagonal Incline Crunch
75	6	Back Extension
89	7	Dumbbell Fly
104	8	Dynaband Side Bend

Twisting Cable Crunch

Target: External obliques, abdominals

Starting Position: Stand or kneel in front of a high pulley and grip a bar with an underhand grip or use a rope (as pictured). Hold the bar so your wrists are close to your ears. Arch your back slightly.

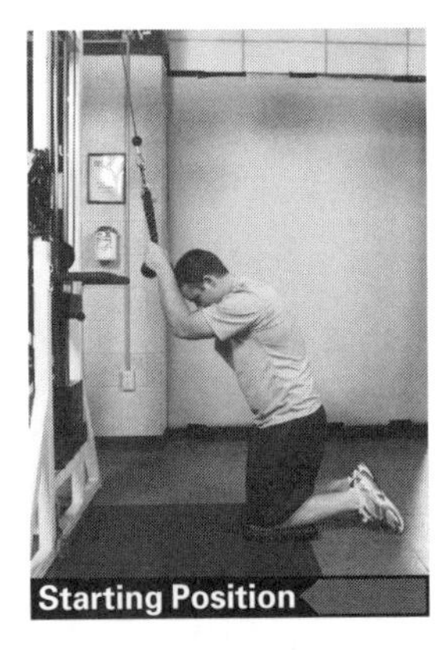
Starting Position

1. Crunch your elbows downward, pivoting at the bottom of your rib cage, and rotate your body to one side. Squeeze hard.

2. Rise up until your back is arched again in the starting position.

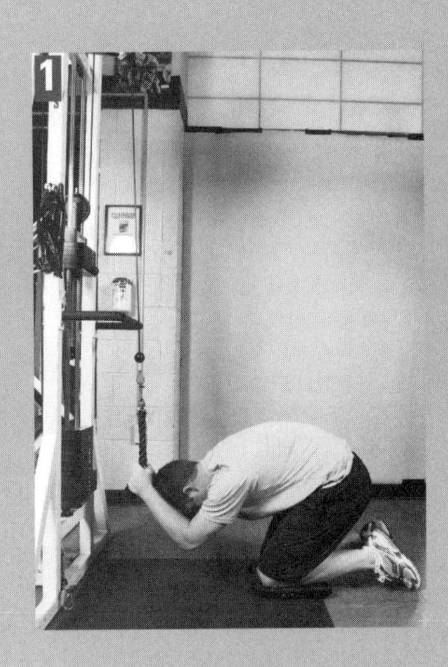
1

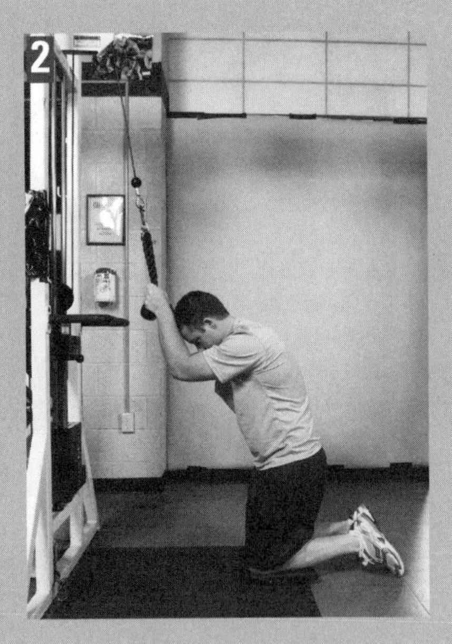
2

Machine Back Extension

Target: Erector spinae

Starting Position: Sit down on the machine and keep your lower back and upper body against the support pads. Tuck your chin in and cross your arms across your chest.

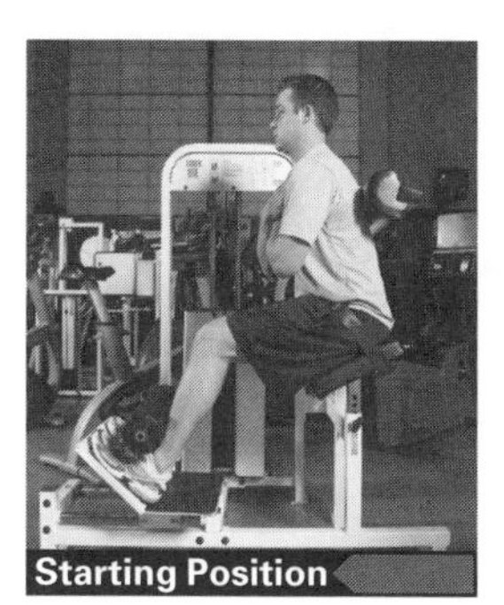
Starting Position

1. Push against the pad until you are reclined. Hold.
2. Slowly return to starting position.

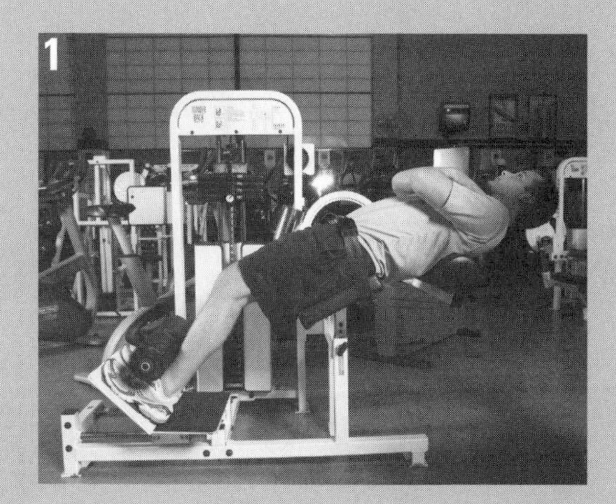
1

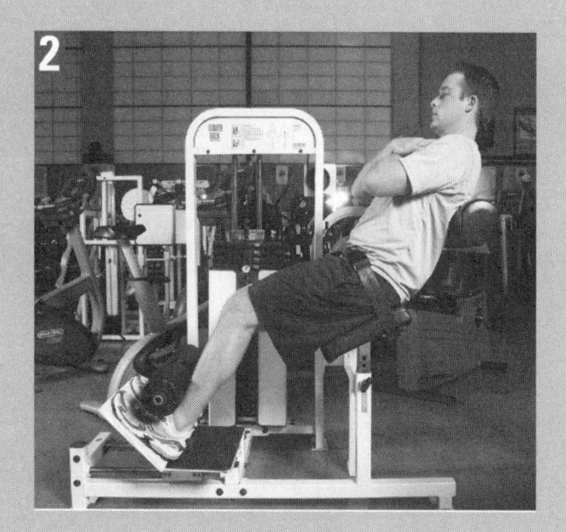
2

Close-Grip Chin-Up

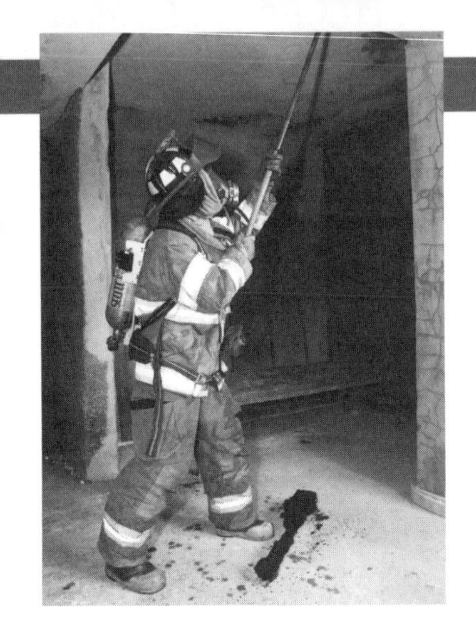

Target: Biceps

Imagine that you're grabbing hold of the ceiling boards and pulling them down.

Starting Position: Grasp the bar with your hands approximately 6 inches apart and your palms facing you. Hang from the bar with your arms fully extended.

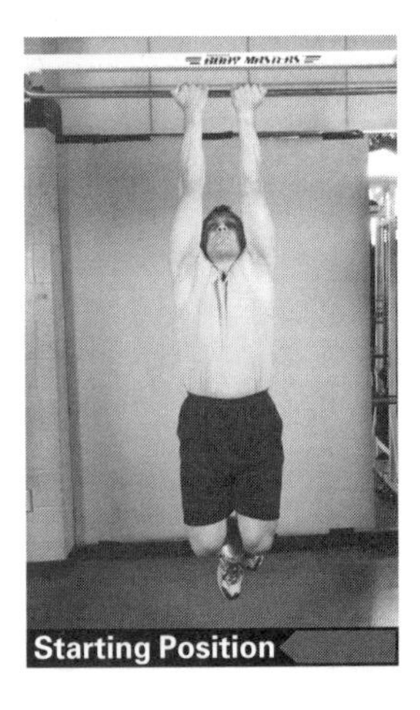
Starting Position

1. Bend your elbows and pull your chest upward toward the bar; hold.
2. Slowly return to starting position.

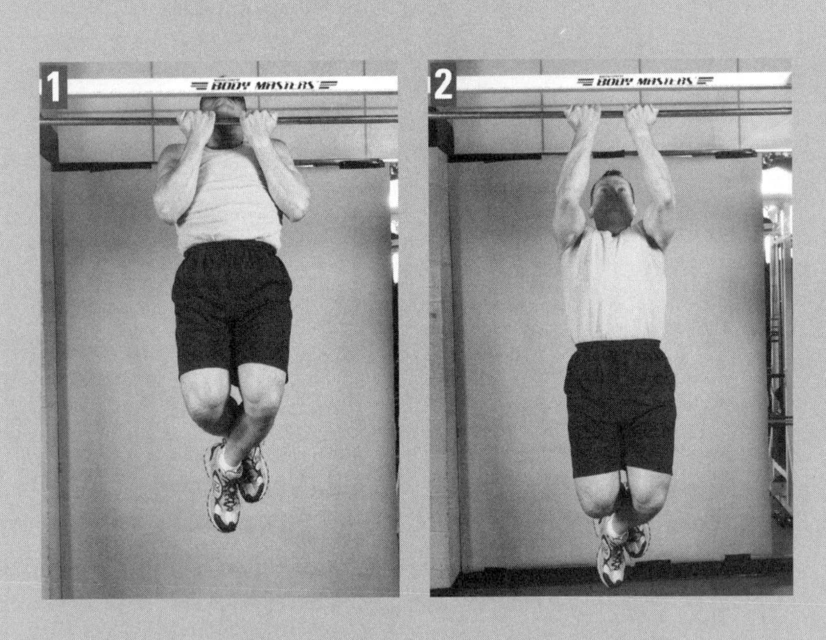

Pull-Up

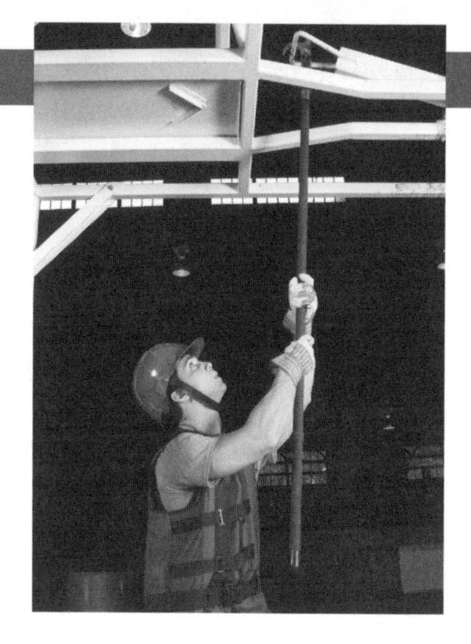

Target: Latissimus dorsi and biceps

Starting Position: Grasp the bar with your hands about shoulder-width apart, palms facing away from you. Hang from the bar with your arms fully extended.

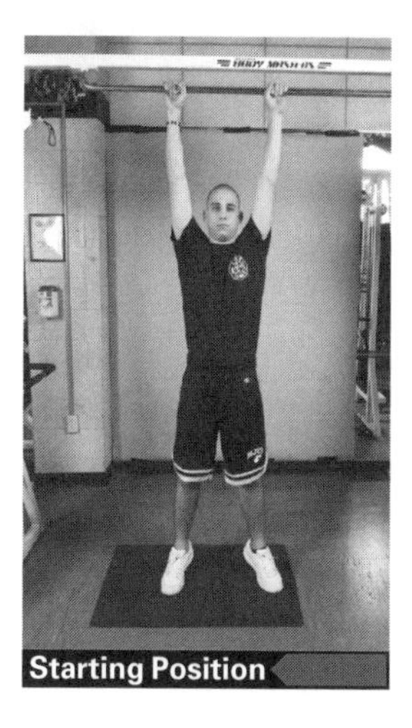
Starting Position

1. Bend your elbows and pull your chest up toward the bar; hold.
2. Slowly return to starting position.

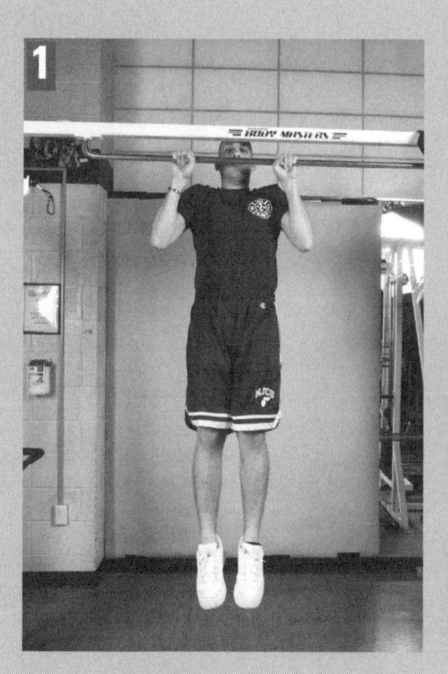
1

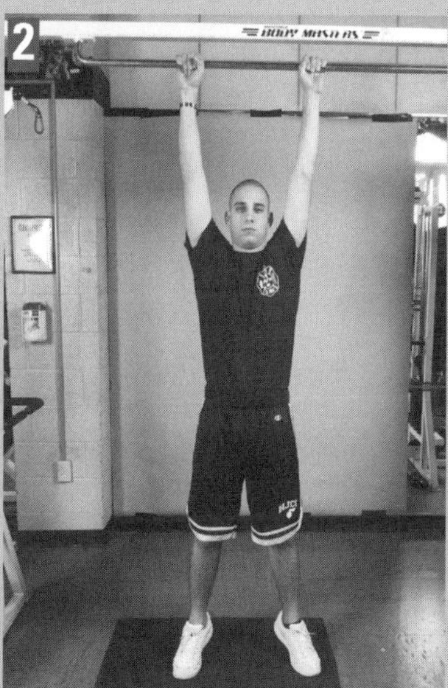
2

Endnotes & Recommended Reading

ENDNOTES

1. Andreachi, M. Personal conversation. 1985
2. Bailey, C. *The Fit or Fat Target Diet.* Boston: Houghton Mifflin Co., 1984.
3. Brosnan, J. Personal conversation. 1986.
4. Burns, J. Personal conversation. 1979.
5. Conte, R. Personal conversation. 1999.
6. De Meersman, R. Personal conversation. 2003.
7. Healey, C. Personal conversation. 1998.
8. Malley, K. S., A. M. Goldstein, T. K. Aldrich, K. J. Kelly, M. Weiden, N. Coplan, M. L. Karwa and D. J. Prezant. "Effects of fire fighting uniform (modern, modified modern and traditional) design changes on exercise duration in New York City firefighters." *Journal of Occupational and Environmental Medicine.* 41:1104-1115. 1999.
9. McArdle, W. D., F. I. Katch and V. L. Katch. *Exercise Physiology: Energy, Nutrition and Human Performance.* 6th ed. Philadelphia: Lea & Febiger, 2007.
10. McLaughlin, J. Personal conversation. 1986.
11. McFadden, P. Personal conversation. 1997.
12. Myerjack, J. Personal conversation. 1992.
13. Pritikin, N. *The Pritikin Program for Diet and Exercise.* New York: Bantam Dell Publishing Group, 1979.
14. Shiraldi, N. Personal conversation. 1985.

RECOMMENDED READING

In an effort to make this book as readable, understandable, enjoyable and useable as possible, we have minimized the length and detail of our explanations, and the use of technical language, data and statistics. If you'd like to gain a better understanding of exercise physiology, training and nutrition, we recommend the following books.

Dave and I were introduced to the work of these authors through the course of our mentoring by two acknowledged masters in the fields of exercise science and applied physiology: Dr. William D. McArdle, Queens College of New York City, and Dr. Ronald E. DeMeersman, Teachers College, Columbia University. The information we have presented was largely obtained through their teachings and from the information provided by the authors of these and other books. Reading **list A** is composed of books that we recommend for those with little or no background in exercise science, training and nutrition. **List B** features books that are more appropriate for individuals with a stronger background in these areas.

List A

Alter, J. *Stretch and Strengthen.* Boston: Houghton Mifflin Company, 1986.

Anderson, B. *Stretching: 20th Anniversary.* Bolinas, California: Shelter Publications, Inc., 2000.

Baechle, T. R. and R. W. Earle. *Weight Training: Steps to Success.* 3rd ed. Champaign, Illinois: Human Kinetics Publishing, 2006.

Bailey, C. *Fit or Fat?* Boston: Houghton Mifflin Company, 1978.

——— *The Fit or Fat Target Diet: The Easiest Plan for Your Best Diet.* Boston: Houghton Mifflin Company, 1989.

Coe, P. *Winning Running: Successful 800m & 1500m Racing and Training.* Wiltshire, England: The Crowood Press, 1996.

Cooper, K. H. *Aerobics Program for Total Well-Being: Exercise, Diet and Emotional Balance.* New York: Bantam Publishing, 1985.

——— *New Aerobics for Women.* New York: Bantam Publishing, 1988.

Daniels, J. *Daniel's Running Formula: Proven Programs 800m to the Marathon.* 2nd ed. Champaign, Illinois: Human Kinetics Publishing, 2005.

Delavier, F. *Strength Training Anatomy.* 2nd ed. Champaign, Illinois: Human Kinetics Publishing, 2006.

——— *Women's Strength Training Anatomy.* Champaign, Illinois: Human Kinetics Publishing, 2003.

Fixx, J. *Jim Fixx's Second Book of Running.* 1st ed. New York: Random House Publishing, 1980.

Galloway, J. *Galloway's Book on Running.* 2nd ed. Bolinas, California: Shelter Publications, 2002.

Henderson, J. *Run Farther, Run Faster.* New York: Collier Books, 1985.

Henderson, J. and H. Higdon. *Running 101: Essentials for Success.* 1st ed. Champaign, Illinois: Human Kinetics Publishing, 2000.

McArdle, W. D., F. I. Katch and V. L. Katch. *Sports and Exercise Nutrition.* 2nd ed. Philadelphia: Lippincott Williams & Wilkins, 2005.

Nokes, T. *Lore of Running.* 4th ed. Champaign, Illinois: Human Kinetics Publishing, 2002.

Oliver, D. and D. Healy. *Athletic Strength for Women.* Champaign, Illinois: Human Kinetics Publishing, 2005.

Ornish, D. *Eat More Weigh Less.* New York: Quill, 2000.

Pritikin, N. *Pritikin Program for Diet and Exercise.* New York: Bantam Dell Publishing Group, 1984.

——— *The Pritikin Promise: 28 Days to a Longer, Healthier Life.* New York: Simon & Schuster Publishing, 1983.

Sandler, D. *Weight Training Fundamentals: A Better Way to Learn the Basics.* Champaign, Illinois: Human Kinetics Publishing, 2003.

Sheehan, G. *Running and Being: The Total Experience.* 20th ed. New Jersey: Second Wind II Publishers, 1998.

Wardlaw, G. M. and A. Smith. *Contemporary Nutrition.* 6th ed. New York: McGraw Hill Publishers, 2004.

Wasser, A. and D. Kimble. *Mastering the CPAT: A Comprehensive Guide.* Clifton Park, New York: Thompson Delmar Learning, 2007.

List B

Astrand, P. O., K. Rodahl, H. A. Dahl and S. Stromme. *Textbook of Work Physiology.* 4th ed. Champaign, Illinois: Human Kinetics Publishing, 2003.

Berne, R. M. *Principles of Physiology.* 2nd ed. Chicago, Illinois: Mosby Year Book Medical Publishers, 1996.

Brody, T. *Nutritional Biochemistry.* 2nd ed. Burlington, Massachusetts: Academic Press, 1999.

Brooks, G. A., T. D. Fahey and K. M. Baldwin. *Exercise Physiology Human Bioenergetics and Its*

Applications. 4th ed. New York: McGraw Hill Publishers, 2004.

Costill, D. and S. Trappe. *Running: The Athlete Within*. Traverse City, Michigan: Cooper Publishing, 2002.

Enoka, R. M. *Neuromechanical Basis of Kinesiology*. 2nd ed. Champaign, Illinois: Human Kinetics Publishing, 1994.

The Fire Service Joint Labor Management Wellness Fitness Initiative. *International Association of Fire Fighters*. International Standard Book Number: 0-942920-36-8, 1999.

The Fire Service Joint Labor Management Wellness Fitness Initiative Candidate Physical Ability Test. *International Association of Fire Fighters*. International Standard Book Number: 0-942920-41-4, 1999.

Fleck, S. and W. J. Kraemer. *Designing Resistance Training Programs*. 2nd ed. Champaign, Illinois: Human Kinetics Publishing, 1997.

Guyton, A. C. and J. E. Hall. *Textbook of Medical Physiology*. 10th ed. Oxford, England: W. B. Saunders Company, 2000.

McArdle, W. D., F. I. Katch and V. L. Katch. *Exercise Physiology: Energy, Nutrition and Human Performance*. 6th ed. Philadelphia: Lippincott Williams & Wilkins, 2006.

——— *Sports & Exercise Nutrition*. 2nd ed. Philadelphia: Lippincott Williams & Wilkins, 2007.

——— *Essentials of Exercise Physiology*. 3rd ed. Philadelphia: Lea & Febiger, 1994.

Powers, S. K. and E. T. Howley. *Exercise Physiology: Theory and Application to Fitness and Performance*. 6th ed. New York: McGraw Hill Publishers, 2007.

Stipanuk, M. H. *Biochemical and Physiological Aspects of Human Nutrition*. 1st ed. Oxford, England: W. B. Saunders Company, 2000.

Tipton, C. *ACSM's Advanced Exercises Physiology*. Philadelphia: Lippincott Williams & Wilkins, 2006.

Wassermann, K., J. E. Hansen, D. Y. Sue, W. W. Stringer and B. J. Whipp. *Principles of Exercise Testing and Interpretation*. 4th ed. Philadelphia: Lippincott Williams & Wilkins, 2004.

Wilmore, J. H., D. Costill and L. W. Kenney. *Physiology of Sport and Exercise*. 4th ed. Champaign, Illinois: Human Kinetics Publishing, 2007.

Index

Any earnings from the sale of this book that may have been directed to Kevin S. Malley will instead be dedicated to a New Jersey City University Foundation educational scholarship fund. The fund honors two members of our faculty/staff, FDNY Firefighter Thomas A. Gardner and FDNY Lieutenant Kevin W. Donnelly, who made the supreme sacrifice on 9/11/01 while operating at the NYC World Trade Center. Tax-deductible contributions may be made payable to the Gardner/Donnelly NJCU Foundation Scholarship and sent to:

NJCU Foundation University Advancement-H321
New Jersey City University
2039 Kennedy Blvd.
Jersey City, New Jersey 07035-1597

For more information, call 201-200-3489.

In Memoriam

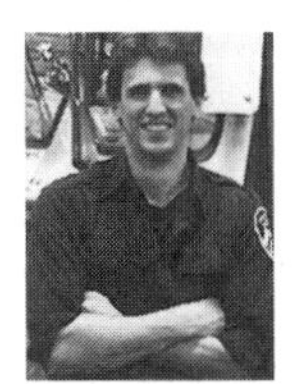

Thomas A. Gardner was a well-educated, intelligent and conscientious person who epitomized the qualities and capacities of a true high-performance firefighter. Working for a number of years in Harlem's Engine Company 59, he established himself as a skilled and incredibly tough nozzleman. Later in his career, Tom utilized his college education in chemistry, working as a member of FDNY's Hazardous Materials Unit 1. Tom excelled in that capacity, and began teaching on the subject of hazardous materials operations nation-wide as well as in the Fire Science Program at New Jersey City University. He was an extraordinary human and great friend, but, more importantly, he was a loving husband and father to his wife Elizabeth and children Christopher and Amy.

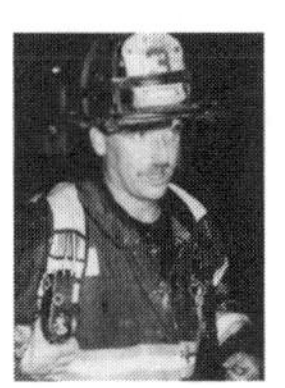

Kevin W. Donnelly was a bright, soft-spoken and highly capable firefighter who worked in Brooklyn's famed "Tin House" (Engine Company 232 & Ladder Company 176) as a firefighter, and then later as an officer in Manhattan's Ladder Company 3. He was an extremely fit marathon runner who used his job skills and courage to perform at the highest level in the field, earning several commendations for his acts of firefighting skill and bravery. He was also very well educated, teaching in New York University's Fire Safety Director Program. In 2000, we had the honor of having Kevin join us at NJCU. He helped to develop and then taught in the NJCU Fire Safety Managers Program. His charismatic personality and giving nature made him as great a teacher as he was a firefighter and fire officer.

About the Contributors

Kevin S. Malley is the chairperson of the fire science department at New Jersey City University. Earning Master's degrees in exercise physiology and applied physiology from Queens College and Teachers College, Columbia University, respectively, he also teaches nutrition and human physiology at the graduate and undergraduate levels. As a member of the New York City Fire Department for more than 22 years, Kevin worked in engine, ladder and special operations units as a firefighter and fire officer. In 1996, he was appointed as the FDNY director of human performance, where he was responsible for the physical conditioning programs of FDNY's firefighter, EMS and civilian personnel. He also served as an FDNY representative working on the International Association of Fire Fighters/International Association of Fire Chiefs (IAFF/IAFC) Joint Labor Management Wellness/Fitness Initiative, Candidate Physical Ability Test and Peer Trainer program. Recently, he contributed to the National Fallen Firefighters Foundation (NFFF) wellness productions *Turnout for Life & Keep Fit for the Fight*, and is researching the influence of circuit-type resistance training on nervous system control of the cardiovascular system in firefighters. A gymnast on SUNY Cortland's championship team in the 1970s, Kevin has since completed more than 20 marathons and won races at distances ranging from the mile to the marathon. Today his physical training happily centers on whatever the season inspires his two children, Kathleen and Kevin, to pursue.

David K. Spierer is currently an assistant professor and director of the human performance laboratory in the division of sports sciences at Long Island University in Brooklyn, New York. He teaches future exercise scientists on topics of exercise testing, instrumentation and clinical exercise pathology. David received his doctorate of education in applied physiology from Teachers College, Columbia University, in 2004. His current research interests involve an investigation of the effects of 12-week circuit weight training on nervous system control of heart rate and blood pressure in firefighters. In addition, he is currently examining the effect of six weeks of core exercise and active isolated stretching on sprint performance. David trains and competes in triathlons and is currently conducting physiological testing on two Olympic hopefuls in track and field. He lives in New York with his wife and two children.

William Wittkop is a professional photojournalistic commercial photographer who has worked for many different companies, organizations and institutions in the NY/NJ metropolitan area for the past 30 years. During the photo shoot, Bill gained a new respect for what it takes to be a firefighter.